BEAUTY MAKEOVER GUIDE

The Helena Rubinstein Library of Beauty
Series editor: Barbara Bonn

Working Woman's Beauty Book
Sharron Hannon

Beauty Makeover Guide
Judith Ross and Susan Acton

Prime of Life Beauty Book
John Foreman
with the Helena Rubinstein Beauty Experts

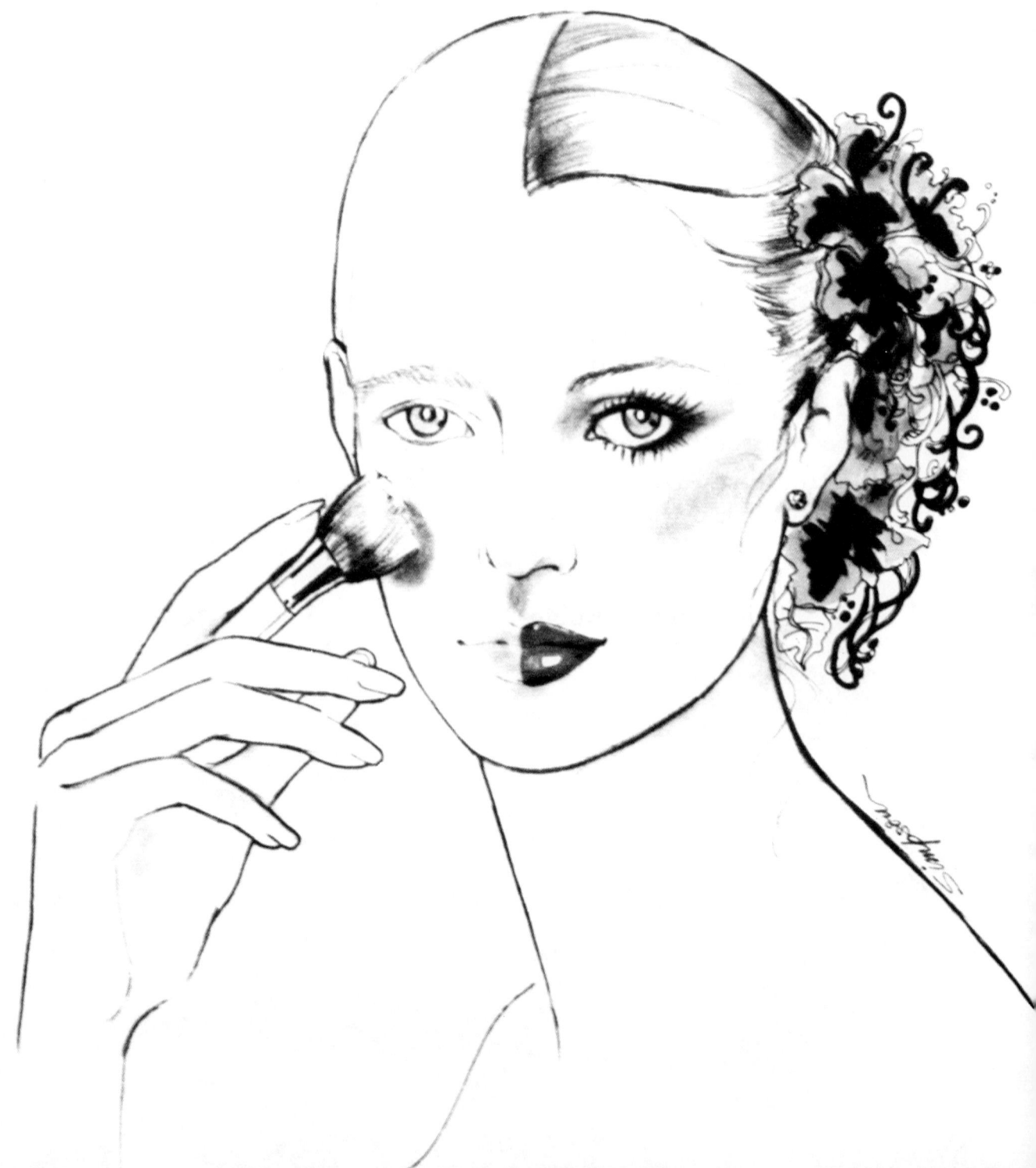

THE **HELENA RUBINSTEIN** LIBRARY OF BEAUTY

BEAUTY MAKEOVER GUIDE

Judith Ross

Susan Acton

with illustrations by
Paula Joseph

STEIN AND DAY/*PUBLISHERS*/ NEW YORK

First published in 1979.
Copyright © 1979 by Helena Rubenstein, Inc.
All rights reserved
Printed in the United States of America
Stein and Day/Publishers/Scarborough House
Briarcliff Manor, N.Y. 10510

Book Design: Michaelis/Carpelis Design

Library of Congress Cataloging in Publication Data

Ross, Judith.
   Beauty makeover guide.

   1. Beauty, Personal. I. Acton, Susan, joint author. II. Title.
RA778.R62   646.7'2   78-19956
ISBN 0-8128-2537-3

CONTENTS

OUTWARD APPEARANCE DOES MATTER	11
ACCENT ON SKIN Determining Skin Type, Allergy Test, Cleaning, Toning, Moisturizing, Facial Masks, Facial Steams, Problems, Weather Care	13
MORE THAN KEEPING CLEAN Baths, Showers, Saving Your Smile, Unwanted Hair, Deodorant, Scent Sense, Forms of Fragrance	30
HOW TO DETERMINE FACIAL SHAPE Oval, Round, Square, Triangle, Inverted Triangle, Diamond	43

FACE FLATTERY	50

Undertoners, Foundation, Highlighter/
Contourer, Concealer, Powder, Liners, Shadows,
Eye Shapes, Mascara, False Lashes, Eyebrows,
Cheek Color, Lips

HIGHLIGHT ON HAIR	93

Hair Type, Care of Hair, Shampoo, Going to a
Hairdresser, Choosing a Hairstyle, Blow-Dry
Techniques, Permanents, Color Problems,
Special Effects

AN IMPORTANT FOCUS	111
ACCENT ON HANDS	113
ACCENT ON FEET	118
ILLUSTRATED MAKEOVERS	122
THE FRAME GAME	128
CONTACT LENSES	133
FASHIONING YOUR WARDROBE	135

BODY TONICS	143

Basic Four, Necessary Nutrients, Healthy/
Unhealthy Foods

BODY TONERS	150
Don't Move, Spot Exercises, Sport Exercises	
WHEN TO SEE A DOCTOR	168
THE RELAXATION EXERCISE	169
SLEEP	169
A WORD ON COSMETIC SURGERY	170
THE RIGHT TIMES	172
PERFECTING NEW TECHNIQUES	177
CONCLUSION	183
Terms to Remember, Readings for Health	

OUTWARD APPEARANCE DOES MATTER

It reflects how you feel about yourself, which in turn influences how others feel about you. If you know you look good and people are responding well to you, self-confidence increases and worries decrease. You are free to enjoy yourself.

Being beautiful, regardless of natural endowments, is a matter of proper health care and the application of the fundamentals of cosmetic techniques. The idea of a beauty makeover is to take what you have and make it look even better, a process that is neither difficult nor time consuming, as we have simplified for you the basic principles that beauty experts depend upon. You can now experiment and improve your image at home. Hair, skin, features, and body have been clearly defined into various types, followed by an explanation of their maintenance and the treatment of problems or flaws. Simply note the descriptions that apply to you, and follow the directions and regimens that correspond to your type. The additional tips will make your makeover even easier.

Whether you seek an answer to a specific beauty problem or want an entirely new look, follow our guidelines. You will definitely notice positive changes in your appearance. It will still be you, but now a more beautiful you.

Remember, it's possible to be healthy and not beautiful, but it's impossible to be beautiful and not healthy. Clear, glowing skin, shining hair, all the components of what we find attractive are dependent upon the general state of our bodies. Therefore, as you work out the best skin-care regimen, the most flattering makeup and hairstyle for yourself, and the most attractive wardrobe, take note of how you maintain your health. Maybe that maintenance schedule needs a makeover, too.

ACCENT ON SKIN

Determining Skin Type

With today's light foundations, even a bad complexion can temporarily look all right. But the ideal use of makeup is to accentuate positive characteristics, not simply cover up flaws. Skin that looks good at all times is a possibility for those who *faithfully* follow a set cleansing and moisturizing routine. The basis of your skin-care program and makeup selection is dependent upon the type of skin you have, so read the following charts and choose those characteristics that match your own. If you put into practice the corresponding cleansing routine for three weeks, you will notice a normalization of your skin's oils, brighter and more even color, and a diminishing number of problems, such as breakouts.

Tips for All Skin Types

- Avoid extreme water temperatures; use warm and cool, instead of hot and cold.
- Wash using your fingers, not a washcloth.
- Dilute astringents and toners by applying them to wet cotton pads before use.
- *Use* moisturizers. Our skins need the protection.
- Do not squeeze blemishes.

NORMAL

CHARACTERISTICS	CLEANSING ROUTINE

CHARACTERISTICS

Soft to the touch

●

Healthy, glowing color

●

Medium pores

●

Translucent quality

●

Makeup does not cake

CLEANSING ROUTINE

Twice Daily

Wash with mild soap or cleanser.

●

Use mild toner.

●

Moisturize.

●

Once Weekly

Use a mildly abrasive agent: cleansing grains or a scrub.

OILY

CHARACTERISTICS	CLEANSING ROUTINE
Excess oil	**Three Times Daily**
•	Wash with mild soap and warm water. Rinse 10 times with warm water, 10 times with cool water.
Shine	
•	
Enlarged or clogged pores	•
•	Use astringent.
Blackheads, whiteheads	•
•	Apply light moisturizer.
Thick skin	•
•	Apply medicated cream on blemishes.*
Frequent breakouts	•
•	**Twice Weekly**
Sallow coloring	Use cleansing grains, buffer, or similar scrubbing agent.

* Black and dark-skinned women: Avoid products with resorcinol in them as this chemical can sometimes stain darkly pigmented skin.

DRY

CHARACTERISTICS	CLEANSING ROUTINE
Skin feels rough	**In the Morning**
●	Use cleanser; tissue off.
Tight feeling	●
●	Moisturize.
Flakes, cracks and chaps easily	●
●	**In the Evening**
Fine lines	Wash with a mild, rinsable cleanser, using only warm water. Rinse 20 times with warm water. Moisturize, especially eye area.
●	
Small pores	
●	●
Skin is thin	**Once Weekly**
●	*Gently* use cleansing grains, buffer, or similar scrubbing agent.
Scaly patches	

COMBINATION

CHARACTERISTICS

Dry skin along cheeks and outer circle of face

●

Oiliness in T zone: forehead, nose, chin

CLEANSING ROUTINE

Twice Daily

Wash with mild soap or liquid cleanser.

●

Apply a *mild* toner to skin.

●

Moisturize, concentrating on dry areas.

●

Apply medicated cream to blemishes.

●

Twice Weekly

Use cleansing grains, buffer, or similar scrubbing agent on oily areas.

PROBLEM

CHARACTERISTICS	CLEANSING ROUTINE
Blemishes, breakouts	**Three Times Daily**
●	Wash hands first.
Acne	●
●	Use medicated cleanser or soap. Rinse 10 times with warm water, 10 times with cool water.
Blackheads, whiteheads	
●	
Pits, scars	●
●	Use a mild toner.
Rashes	●
	Moisturize.
	●
	Apply medicated cream where needed.
	●
	Once Weekly
	Use cleansing grains, buffer, or similar scrubbing agent.

SENSITIVE

CHARACTERISTICS

Redness, flushing

•

Rashes

•

Quick reactions to skin products

CLEANSING ROUTINE

Twice Daily

Use a fluid or cream cleanser; wipe off with cotton balls.

•

Use a very mild, diluted toner.

•

Apply light moisturizer.

•

Use hypoallergenic products.

If you are still unsure about your type of skin, try this:

Ten minutes after washing your face, press a piece of tissue paper or linen blotting paper (ask for this at your drugstore) against your nose and forehead. If there's a big oil spot, your skin is oily. If not, wait 15 minutes and press again. A big spot showing up now means you have normal skin. And if a spot doesn't show up for half an hour or more, your skin is dry.

How does your face feel after you wash it with soap and water?

Feels fine? Your skin is either normal or oily.

●

Feels dry in some sections? You have combination skin.

●

Hurts to smile? You have dry skin.

It might help you to copy the proper routine onto a 3-by-5 card and tape it to the bathroom wall until the regimen has become a habit.

Allergy Test

Women with sensitive skin or a history of allergin reactions should give themselves the "allergy test" before using a new product. Rub a small amount of the substance in question on a clean spot of the inner arm. Cover it with a bandage, and 24 hours later check to see if the skin has become red, swollen, or pimply. No reaction usually means it is safe, but particularly sensitive skin should be retested.

●

Skin care, regardless of type, is divided into three steps: cleansing, toning, and moisturizing. The frequency of their use differs; their application does not. The pull of gravity or going against the grain of delicate facial muscles may cause premature sagging or wrinkles; so in any facial procedure, follow these directionals, moving in a gentle manner with easy pressure.

Before cleansing entire face, eye makeup should be removed. No cleansing creams or homemade lotions will dissolve eye makeup as quickly as a commercial product.

Choose an oil-free or oil-based remover, and do the operation very delicately by stroking on the remover with fingertips, waiting a few seconds, and then blotting it off with a tissue or pressed cotton pad.

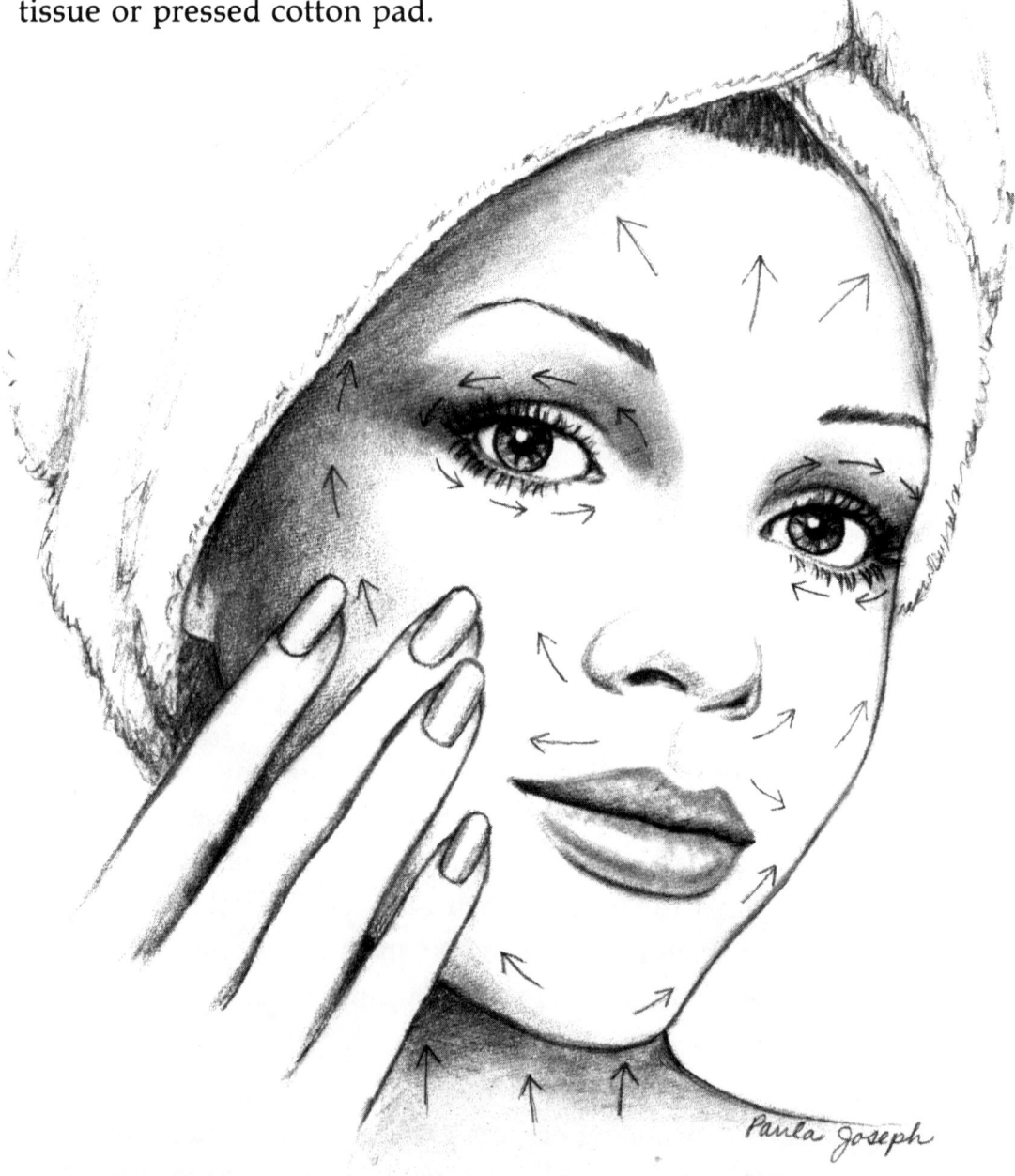

Cleaning

CLEAN to remove makeup, wash off dirt, and open pores so oils can be removed.

If you choose a cleanser, follow the directions. If you select soap and water, lather well and apply to face. Wash gently, please. Let the soap do the work for you. Now rinse, rinse, rinse, first in warm water, then cool. Pat your face dry with a clean towel. Some skin specialists maintain that only soap can thoroughly clean your face, while just as many say soap is too harsh for any skin type. Give cleansers a fair trial, but if soap and water are the only things that make your skin feel clean, go ahead and use them. Be certain that the soap is formulated for your skin type. Cleansers, liquid or cream, are clearly labeled as to which type of skin they're suitable for. Soaps are not, so consult this chart before purchasing your next bar:

TYPE of SOAP

DRY OR SENSITIVE SKIN	NORMAL OR COMBINATION SKIN	OILY OR PROBLEM SKIN
Superfatted	Glycerin	Detergent-based
Low alkaline, creamy Soaps with moisturizers	Castile Transparent	Medicated Transparent

Toning

TONE with specially formulated lotions to close pores, remove dead cells, and restore proper pH balance to skin.

Astringents are generally used for oilier skins, with fresheners and toners used for normal to dry types. Consult with a salesperson to ensure purchasing the proper formula for your skin type. Avoid any with too great an alcohol content. Women with dry skin are better off with fresheners that have no alcohol added at all.

Moisturizing

MOISTURIZE to replenish natural oils, seal in moisture, and protect skin from elements.

Moisturizers are so named because they have humectant qualities, meaning they are able to hold moisture on the surface of the skin and therefore prevent our own valuable moisture from evaporating. Immediately after your face is washed and toned, apply the moisturizer, keeping in mind facial directionals, so that as much moisture as possible will be retained on the skin. Body lotions are not moisturizers; they're thicker, and the oils that compose them will not permit skin to breathe, so don't use them on your face. Formulas have been varied to accommodate areas of the face that are drier than others, such as the throat or eye area. All women should use a moisturizer.

Tips

- Dab moisturizer onto face with a paintbrush if you cannot master a delicate touch with your fingers.
- Moisturize V-area of chest, as well as neck and throat.

Facial Masks

A weekly mask is a great refresher and does much to revitalize your face by stimulating circulation and imparting a natural glow. Clay masks are best for oily skin; moisturizing masks for dry and sensitive skin; and peel-off masks for normal or combination types.

1. Apply the solution to a clean face, avoiding eye area.
2. Keep yourself as expressionless as possible for 15 minutes.
3. Splash off with cool water.
4. Finish with toner and moisturizer.

Facial Steams

A facial steam is the best deep cleanser, because it opens the pores and allows accumulated grime to come to the surface. We recommend it only twice a month, as the steam can dehydrate the skin. Always start with a clean face.

1. Heat a pot of water to boiling.
2. Pour water into large bowl, and hold face a foot above water, keeping eyes shut.

3. Use a towel draped over your head to trap steam.

4. Steam for no longer than eight minutes (or less if you become uncomfortable).

5. Wash face thoroughly; apply toner and moisturizer.

Problems

Here are the six most common skin problems:

PROBLEM: Acne
SYMPTOMS: Persistent breakouts, blackheads, whiteheads, cysts, pimples

TREATMENT: See a doctor no matter how old you are. Keep hands off! Follow our skin-care regimen for problem skin. Use an oil blotter before applying water-based foundation. Use medicated skin-care products. Use a touch stick (a tube of medicated lotion) on pimples, and absorb excess oil with an oil-blotter stick. Improve circulation by exercising, getting fresh air and sunshine, and eating well. Keep hair clean and off the face day and night. Change pillowcase daily.

PROBLEM: Allergy
SYMPTOMS: Itching, bumps or hives, sudden redness, swelling
TREATMENT: See a doctor, especially if condition is serious or persistent. Try to discover what is bothering your skin by eliminating a different skin-care product each week.

PROBLEM: Discoloration

SYMPTOMS: Loss of pigment, brown or reddish blotches of color, brown spots

TREATMENT: See a doctor. Do not attempt to correct discoloration with bleach (this goes for freckles as well). Use a sunscreen. If you're taking birth control pills or medication of any kind, be sure to describe your problem to the doctor who prescribed the medicine.

PROBLEM: Excessive dryness

SYMPTOM: Very dry, flaky, irritated skin

TREATMENT: Apply lots of body lotion to body skin, moisturizer to face skin. Avoid acne medication or water pills. Drink lots of water. Keep a humidifier going in the house. Stay out of the sun and chlorinated pools. Use an oil-based foundation.

PROBLEM: Broken capillaries.

SYMPTOMS: Spidery red or purplish veins

TREATMENT: Keep water temperature for washing from extremes. Avoid exposure to very cold or very warm weather. Don't scrub the area. Don't drink alcoholic beverages. If foundation or body makeup doesn't cover the area and it's a source of embarrassment to you, consult a doctor. The veins can sometimes be removed.

PROBLEM: Wrinkles and lines

SYMPTOMS: Previously smooth skin develops wrinkles and fine lines

TREATMENT: Follow skin-care and general health-care regimens. Always use facial directionals. Use moisturizers. Use a sunscreen if you must be out in the sun. Use a night cream before bedtime. Keep a tube of moisturizer with you for instant use. Give up smoking. Accept the fact that some wrinkles and lines are inevitable as you age.

Notice how most of our treatments include the words "see a doctor"? Assuming that you follow general good health rules and a skin-care regimen such as we have outlined, these problems should not exist. If they do, don't take these problems lightly. Consult a physician.

Weather Care

Cold, wind, heat, sun. There's an endless list of wolves outside our door waiting to destroy our skin and general good feeling. The key word here is *protection* from these harsh environmental factors.

WINTRY WEATHER PROTECTION

Slather yourself with body lotions, hand creams, eye creams and chapsticks lavishly and nonstop. Switch to a superfatted soap and rich bath oil for the bath. Use lotion instead of soap to shave your legs. The sun isn't very strong during the winter, but if you plan to be outside longer than 20 minutes, wear a sun lotion and a lipstick with sun-guard. Add moisture to your house by using a humidifier or leaving pots of water scattered about. And, of course, dress warmly.

SUMMER PROTECTION

Keep cool by drinking lots of liquids, splashing cool water on your face and back of the neck, taking tepid (not cold) showers and walking nude around the house if possible. Keep body lotions in the refrigerator and use them frequently but not so liberally as in the winter.

The sun causes wrinkles. Black-skinned or white-skinned, you must protect yourself with either sunblocks, which totally block out harmful rays, or sunscreens, which permit some rays to reach your skin.

TO TAN SAFELY

1. Start off slowly with a maximum of 15 minutes' exposure on the first couple of days.
2. Never sun during the noon-till-3-p.m. hours.
3. Apply lots of sun protection, remembering the soles of the feet and area around the eyes.
4. Reapply sun protection every time you come out of the water.
5. Don't depend on clothing, hats, or beach umbrellas to shield you from the sun.
6. If you do get burned, take a cool bath with added cider vinegar and apply a benzocaine preparation afterward. If the burn is very painful or blisters, see a doctor.

MORE THAN KEEPING CLEAN

Baths

TOOLS:
- A thick, clean towel
- A long-handled brush for back scrubbing
- A headband, shower cap, or clip to hold back your hair
- A clean washcloth or sponge
- A loofah (a natural spongelike skin stimulator)
- The proper soap (refer to skin-care section)
- Nail brush
- Pumice stone
- A plastic inflatable pillow

If you've been concentrating only on the cleansing aspect of a bath, then you're not making full use of your time spent in the tub, for bathtime is the most productive part of a beauty regimen, allowing time for a luxurious beauty treatment as well as for thorough cleansing from top to toe.

Before bathing, remove your makeup as directed in the skin-care section and wash your face at the sink. A separate wash is necessary, because facial skin requires gentle attention, milder soaps or cleansers, and clean, clear rinse water.

Run water into the tub, avoiding excessive temperatures, as extremes of hot or cold are harmful to the skin. Lightly cream rough edges (elbows, knees, feet) and dry spots (hands, eyes, neck) before entering tub. Now select the type of bath you want, and add the necessary ingredients:

OILS moisturize. Use baby oil, commercial products.

HERBS soothe. Use mint, eucalyptus, pine, commercial products.

MINERALS stimulate and tone skin. Use salt, Epsom salts, commercial products.

KITCHEN WONDERS. Baking soda: A handful soothes skin.
Cider vinegar: 1/3 cup restores pH balance.
Powdered milk: 1/3 cup smooths skin.

Once in, *relax*. Take a deep breath, lie back, supporting your head on the inflated pillow, and just float. Shut your eyes, shut off the world for a few minutes, and feel tensions melt, muscles relax. Next, sit up and scrub your body all over with the loofah (scrub only your rough edges if your skin is dry) to slough off dead skin and bring blood back to the surface. Concentrate on rough edges. Brush your fingernails, toenails, and back with brushes and soap. Rub the pumice stone on calluses. Now lather up well, and swirl your washcloth or sponge around your body in circular motions.

Rinse off first by using tub water and then fresh water, either from the faucet or shower. Step out, dry, and immediately apply body lotion, from your neck to the soles of your feet; the lotion acts as a moisture sealant. Now dust powder all over, and see if you don't already feel like your beauty makeover is working.

Tips

- Rub skin briskly with the rough side of the towel to stimulate.
- Pat skin gently with the smooth side of the towel, if you want to remain relaxed.
- Don't remain in the tub too long, especially if your body is dry; water dehydrates.
- Have a shower caddy to hold all your equipment.
- To keep bath water as clean as possible, don't shave legs or underarms in the tub. Do it while showering.

Showers

Showers are preferred by many women because they are quicker, more conservative in water use, and invigorating. Being a woman doesn't mean you must take a bath every day; two or three baths a week, with showers on the alternate days, are sufficient to keep you clean and fresh.

Showerheads have become more than just water dispensers; their various patterns can be altered from wide, soft sprays to powerful, concentrated jets, so that you can relax, massage or stimulate your skin as desired. While the variety of ingredients that can be added to a bath are excluded from a shower, you can still turn it into a beauty treatment by taking advantage of the assortment of bath gels that stimulate or moisturize. Follow the same procedure as for a bath; that is, wash face first, cream your body's rough edges and dry spots, run warm (not too hot or cold) water, and enter. Get wet and lather well. To give the soap a chance to do its job, stand away from the shower stream until you've completed your washing. Step back under the water and rinse thoroughly. Dry, and apply lotion and powder over the body.

Saving Your Smile

Teeth are the sparkle of your smile as well as a vital tool in the digestion process. A beautiful smile can cover a multitude of faults, so it's worth the effort to protect it.

Your part in tooth care consists of morning and evening brushing, with a thorough flossing at night. They are of equal importance, as brushing cleans the teeth's surfaces, while only flossing can extract particles from the narrow spaces between teeth that the brush cannot reach.

TO BRUSH

1. Use a soft, nylon-bristled brush. Have one brush for the morning, another for night use. in order to give each brush a chance to dry and help prevent bacterial formation.
2. Wet brush and apply a small amount of toothpaste or tooth powder.
3. Gently brush surfaces of teeth, moving only in the direction of the teeth's growth, never back and forth.
4. Rinse mouth and brush thoroughly.
5. Keep brush in open air to avoid bacterial growth.

TO FLOSS

1. Break off 15 to 20 inches of unwaxed floss from container.
2. Wind ends around fingers till only a few inches are left between fingers.
3. Insert floss between teeth, and gently slide it up and down against the side of each tooth from the very top to the bottom.
4. Check with your dentist to be certain you are using the right technique.
5. Don't skip this nightly ritual. It's as necessary as brushing.

Several times a week manually massage your gums. Pretend your finger is a toothbrush, and "brush" your gums. This stimulates circulation and aids in your preventive treatment.

A healthy mouth shouldn't smell foul; bad breath is an indicator of disease, so see your doctor if this is a consistent problem. Mouthwashes do little harm or little good. Their use is a matter of personal preference.

Now that dentists have incorporated preventive medicine into their treatment procedures, the chances of losing your teeth have decreased greatly. At the office, the dentist can slow down or stop the development of diseases, such as dental caries (cavities) or pyorrhea (gum disease) before they become serious, painful problems. Only a professional cleaning done twice a year without fail can thoroughly remove plaque, the sticky, white substance that builds up on teeth and harbors bacteria.

Tips

- Try baking soda instead of toothpaste for a refresher.
- Forget your toothbrush? Use a washcloth.
- Keep a spare toothbrush and extra dental floss in your purse.

Unwanted Hair

Unwanted hair can be dealt with in a variety of ways. You can bleach it, shave it off, pull it off, or burn it off, either with electricity or chemicals. This harsh way of describing hair removal is really to remind you to *be careful*.

If you shave, make sure the razor is clean and sharp. Don't use an electric razor near water. Give yourself an allergy test before using any chemicals. Make certain wax isn't too hot before application. And go to a certified professional for any permanent removal.

Now choose your weapon:

RAZOR SHAVING. A fast, easy method resulting in smooth skin, which is quickly replaced in a day or two with a stubbly growth. Good for legs and underarms and best done in the shower.

ELECTRIC RAZOR. Probably the easiest method of all. Resultant removal isn't so close to the skin as you might desire, but the procedure is easily repeated and takes only a minute or so. Good for legs and underarms.

BLEACHING. Mild bleaches have been formulated specifically for unwanted hair. Follow directions, and these hairs should become very light and unnoticeable. This is the best way to deal with the problems of facial hair short of permanent removal; other methods result in a stubbly growth that is quite masculine in appearance.

DEPILATORIES. Creamy solutions that melt the hair directly below the skin. You merely apply, wait for a few minutes and remove. Because the chemicals involved are strong, you must give yourself an allergy test before their use. Good for legs, stomach, chest. How long a depilatory lasts depends on the product and the individual.

WAXING. A procedure in which warm wax is applied to an area, allowed to cool, then pulled off, carrying the hair practically down to the root with it. This relatively long-lasting procedure is obviously not painless. Good for legs.

ELECTROLYSIS is the insertion of a very fine needle into the hair root through which is sent a tiny destructive electrical current. A low regrowth rate, combined with the time it takes to remove each hair make the process time-consuming and therefore costly. Advantage: It is permanent. Good for facial, chest, and stomach hair.

DEPILATRON, like electrolysis, is a permanent method that kills hair at the roots. The electric current is sent down the hair shaft to the root via special tweezers. It is less uncomfortable than electrolysis, because the skin is not pierced, but it takes longer and is just as expensive. Good for facial and chest hair.

Tips
- Rinse depilatories off in the shower.
- Shave in the direction of hair's growth if your skin is sensitive.
- Don't remove hair from arms. If they are really as hairy as you think, try bleaching.
- For those few embarrassing hairs on the chest, also try bleaching. If you cannot tolerate the bleach, pluck them out.

Deodorant

Perspiration is the skin's natural cooling process. The odor associated with it is caused by bacteria, not by the wetness itself. The amount you perspire is influenced by emotional stress, heat, and physical exertion.

Perspiration may be controlled with a deodorant, an antiperspirant, or talcum powder. Whether in stick, roll-on, cream, spray, or powder form, they all help to control wetness and odor to some degree. A deodorant primarily controls the odor, while an antiperspirant checks the wetness. Most people prefer deodorants. If you don't perspire much, you may find that a sprinkle of talcum powder or baking soda is enough control for you. If you perspire heavily, you may need an antiperspirant. Excessive perspiration is a condition that should be checked by a doctor.

The best time to apply your deodorant is a few minutes after a bath or shower in order to prevent odors before they have a chance to begin.

Tips

- Never use a deodorant or antiperspirant immediately after shaving under the arms.
- Wash stale deodorants or antiperspirants away before reapplying.

Scent Sense

Fragrance is an undeniable asset in any beauty routine. It has the power to lift and lighten the spirit and complete the total feeling of freshness. Choose discriminately. Your best friend's favorite perfume may be disastrous for you since individual body chemistries differ. Knowing the characteristics of the various types of scent may help you select a suitable one for you.

TYPE	CHARACTERISTICS	AROMAS
FLORAL	Sweet • Fresh	Blends of flowers • Single flower scent
WOODSY	Woodsy • Mossy	Ferns • Herbs • Forest blends

SPICY	Long-lasting	Vanilla or ginger
	•	•
	Pungent	Oranges
	•	•
	Distinctive	Carnations
ORIENTAL	Intriguing	Sandalwood
	•	•
	Exotic	Musk
	•	•
	Warm	Incense

MODERN　　　Sophisticated　　　Combination of all above

•

Sparkling

•

Rich

Forms of Fragrance

Scents come in many forms. Body warmth releases the true essence of all of them, so use them right after a bath while your skin is still warm. Apply fragrance at these points in order to create a lingering effect:

At the temples

•

Behind the ears

•

Nape of neck

•

Base of throat

•

Between the breasts

●

Inside of wrists

●

Behind the knees

●

Inside of ankles

NOTE: Never apply any fragrance to the genital area because of the risk of infection.

Perfume is the strongest and longest lasting form of fragrance. Cologne and eau fraiche are less concentrated forms.

COLOGNE. The most popular form of fragrance, because it's less expensive and can be used freely without fear of becoming overpowering. Cologne can be found in aerosol, stick, solid, or roll-on form, as well as liquid.

EAU FRAICHE or TOILET WATER. Less concentrated than cologne but does not have the staying power that cologne has, so use it generously.

SACHETS. Lacy little bags to scent clothing in drawers or closets. Cream sachets are also popular and should be applied directly to the skin.

Scent has been added to body lotions, bath oils, dusting powders, soaps, candles, and even stationery. Enjoy using more than one form of your favorite fragrance in order to enhance its effect.

Tips

- Try a few drops of your favorite cologne in the rinse water of your lingerie, hairbrushes, and combs.
- Never try on more than two or three scents in one shopping trip. Your sense of smell can't handle more than that.
- Keep your scent in the refrigerator for a cool bracer.
- Don't wear perfume when sunbathing; the combination of sun and perfume can cause your skin to have an allergic reaction.
- Keep all forms out of direct sunlight, as it destroys their fragrance.

HOW TO DETERMINE FACIAL SHAPE

You will save invaluable time and money by determining your facial shape before attempting any beauty makeovers. You cannot separate the shape of your face from selecting and applying your makeup or from selecting complementary hairstyles and eyeglasses.

FACIAL SHAPES

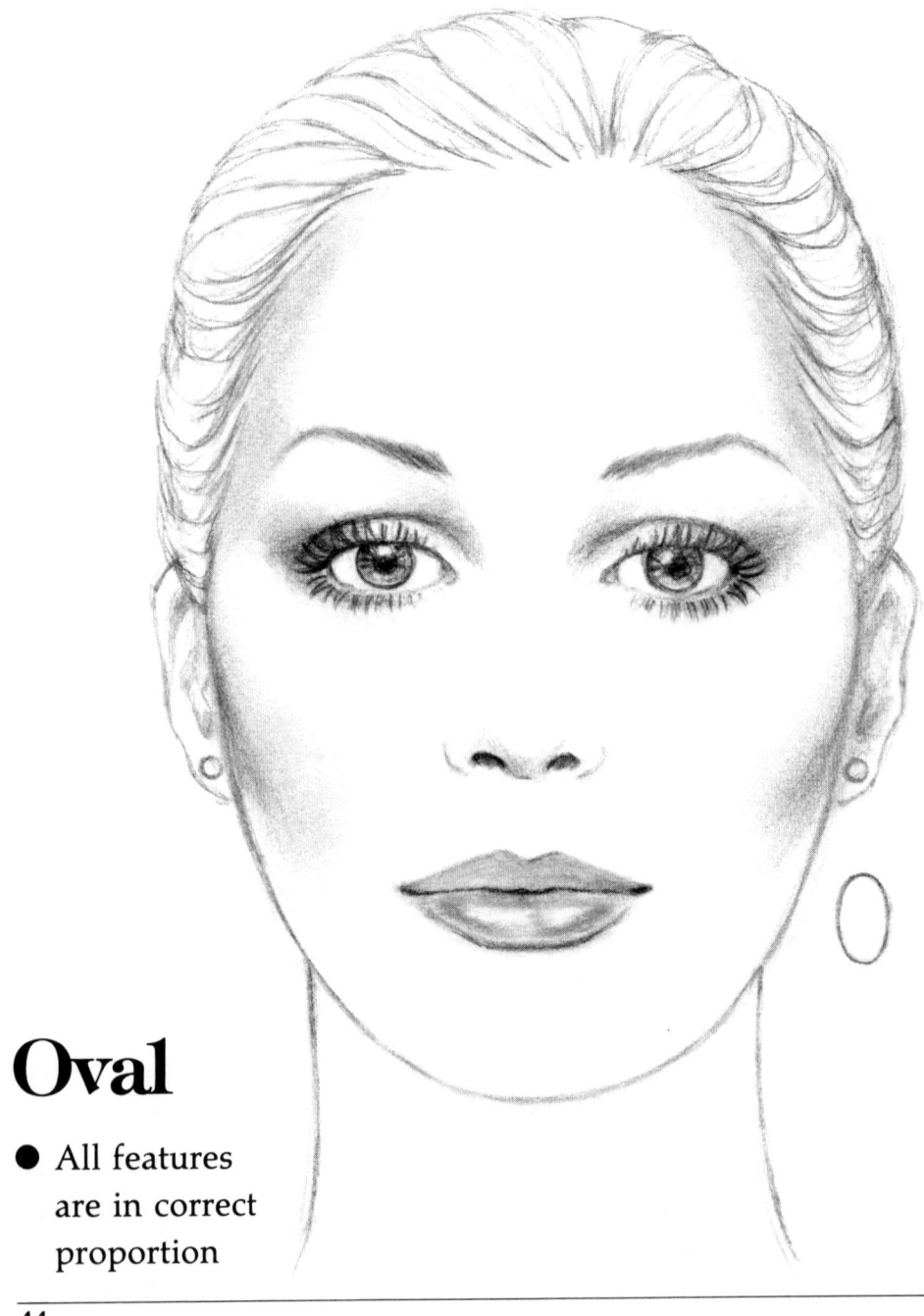

Oval

- All features are in correct proportion

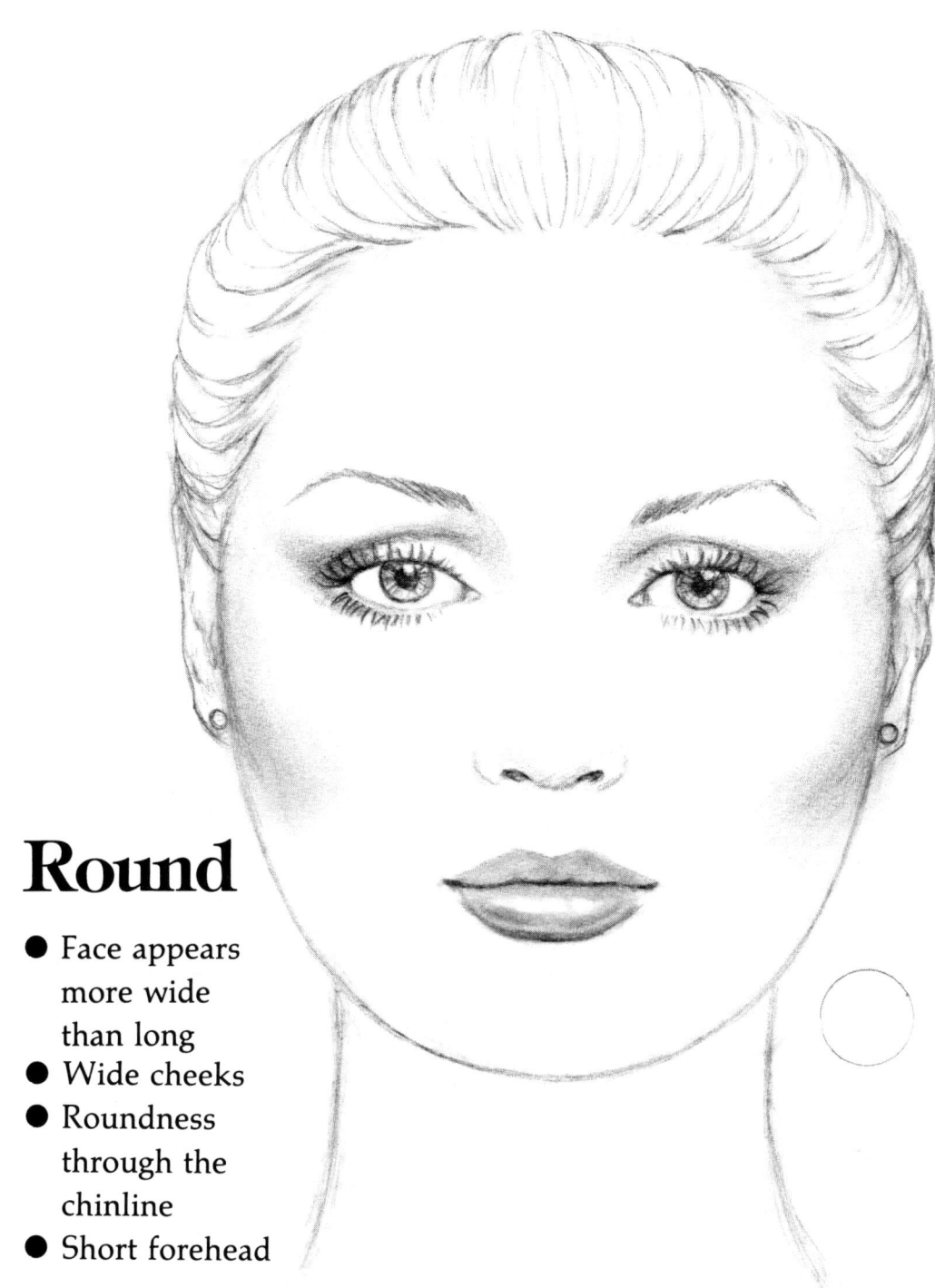

Round

- Face appears more wide than long
- Wide cheeks
- Roundness through the chinline
- Short forehead

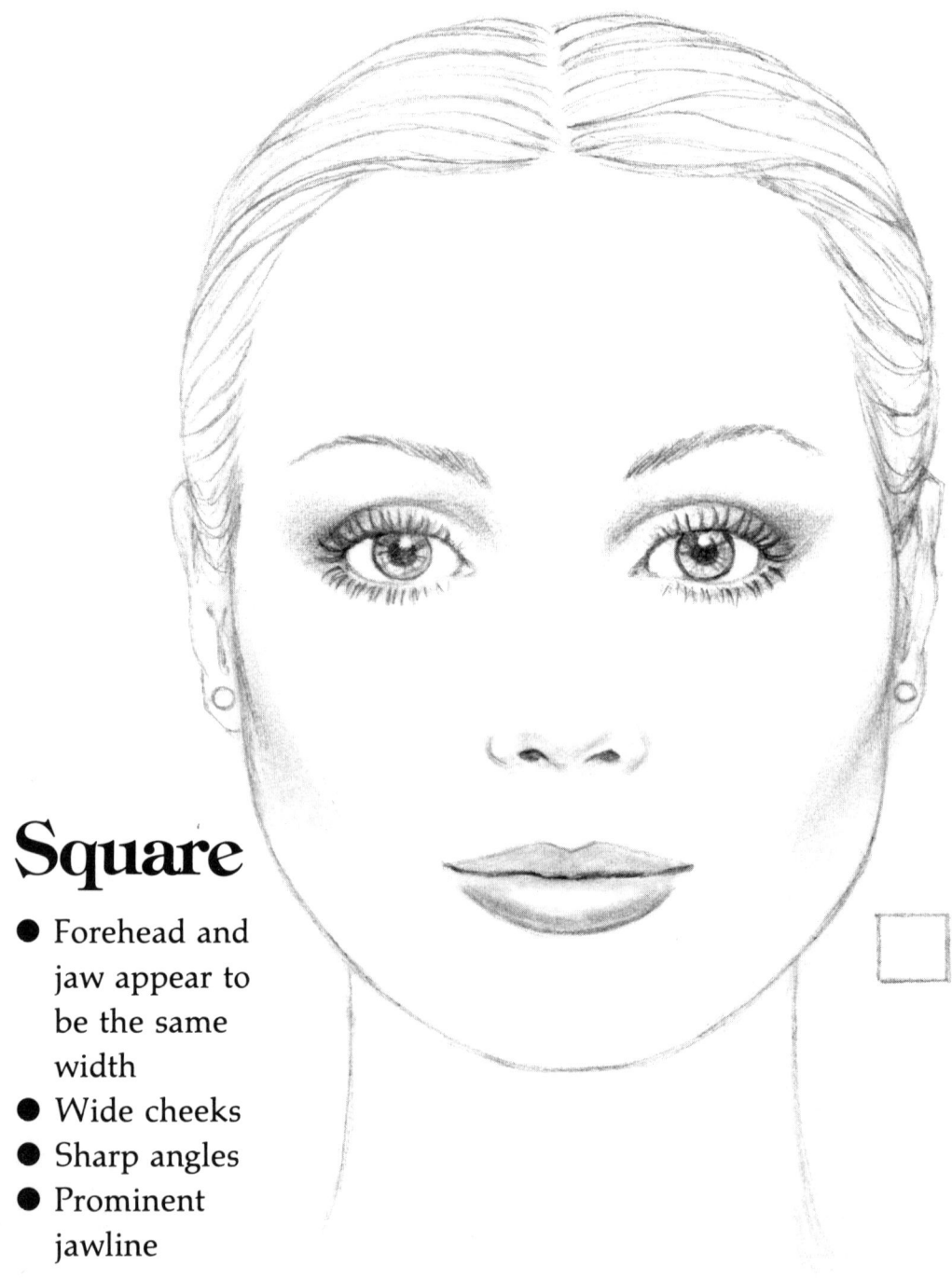

Square

- Forehead and jaw appear to be the same width
- Wide cheeks
- Sharp angles
- Prominent jawline

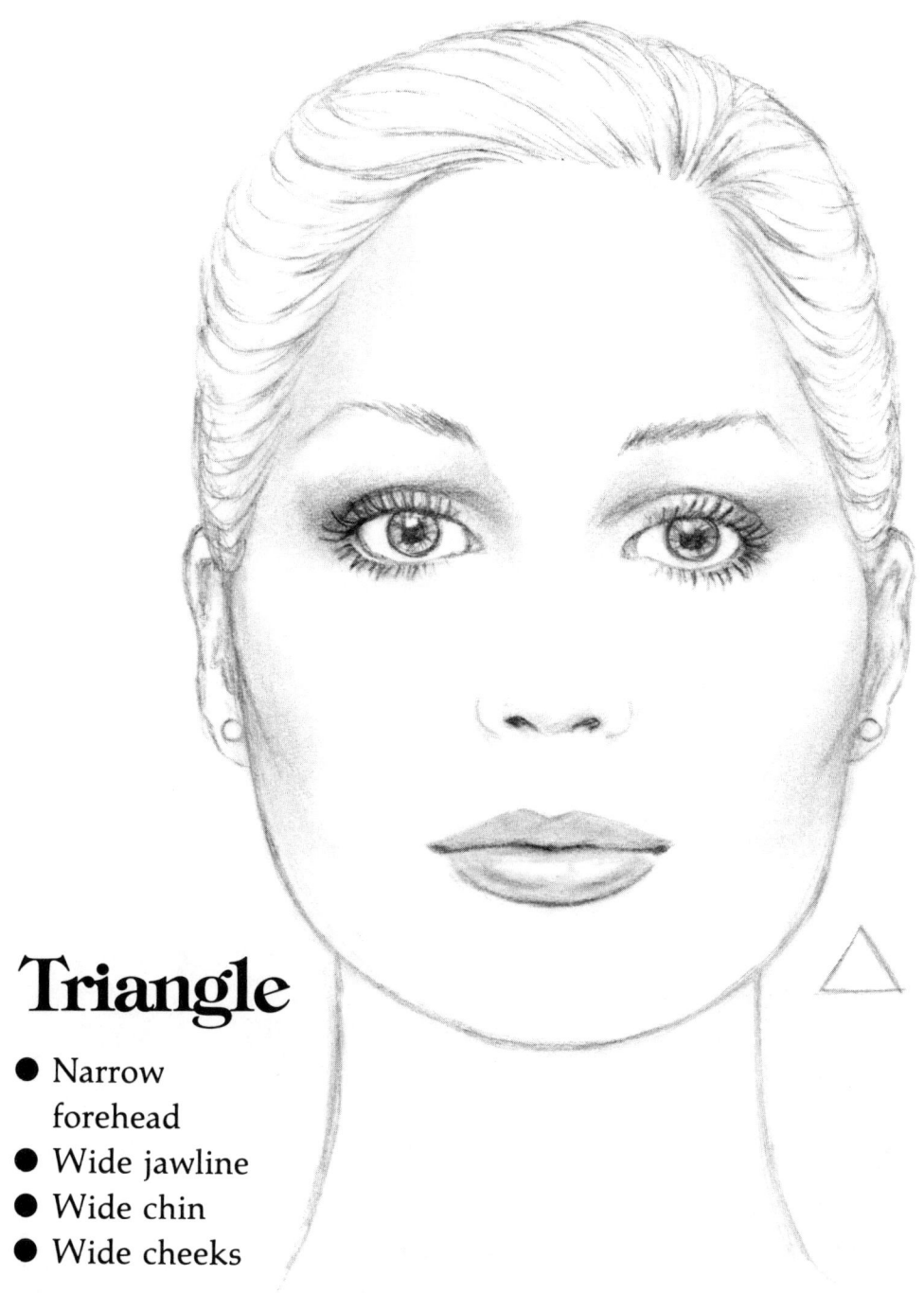

Triangle

- Narrow forehead
- Wide jawline
- Wide chin
- Wide cheeks

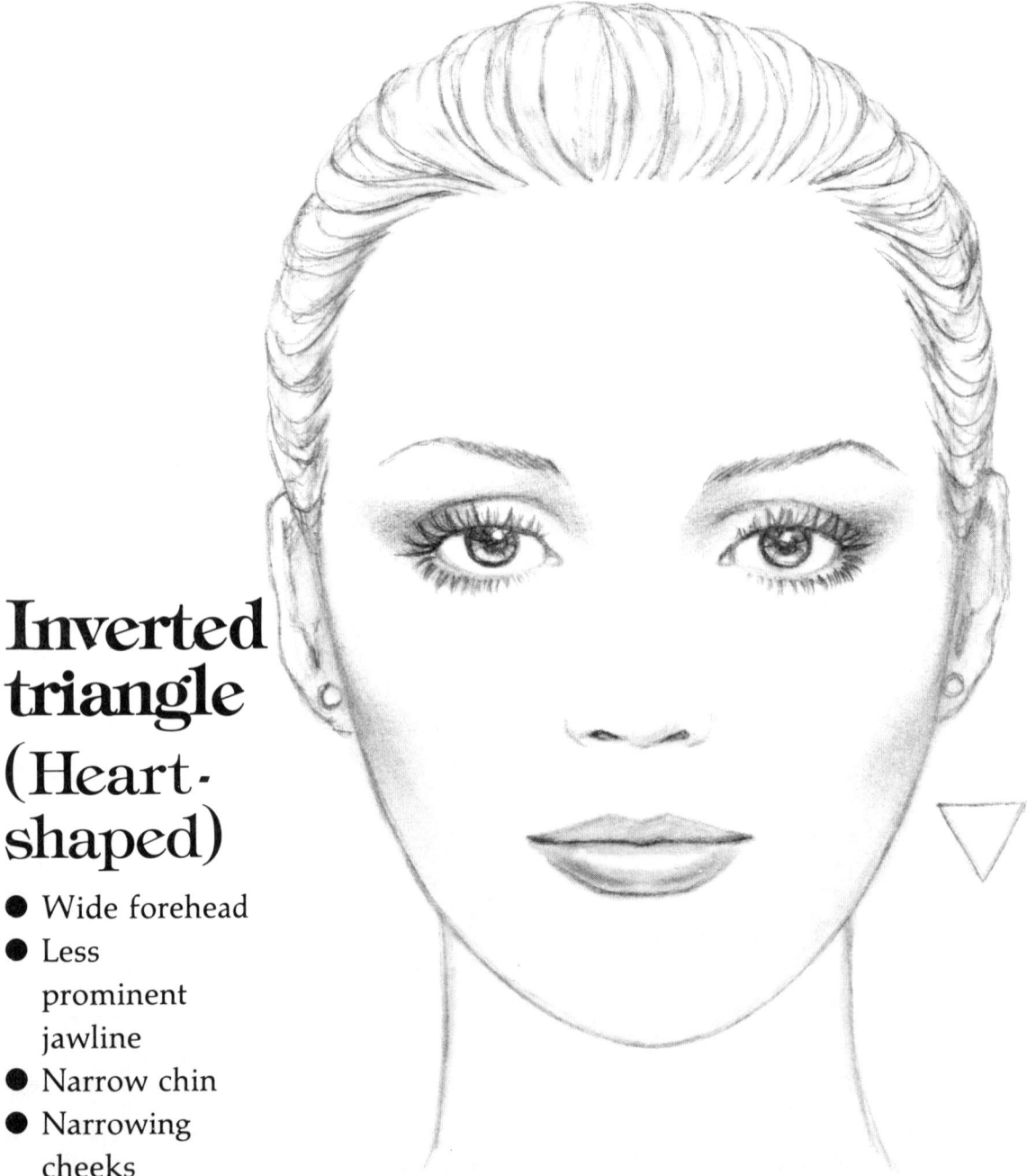

Inverted triangle (Heart-shaped)

- Wide forehead
- Less prominent jawline
- Narrow chin
- Narrowing cheeks

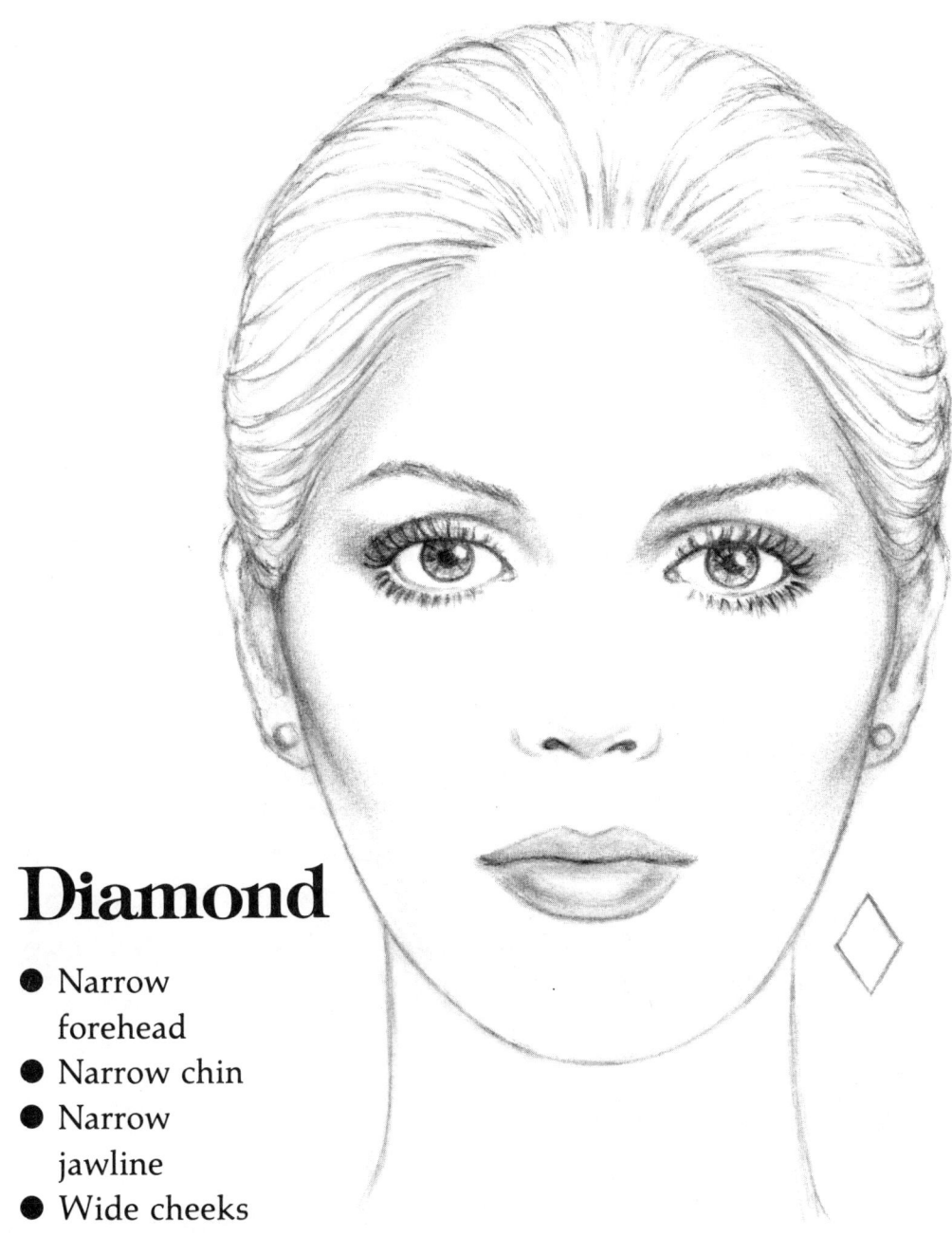

Diamond

- Narrow forehead
- Narrow chin
- Narrow jawline
- Wide cheeks

Tips
- Under bright lights, in front of your mirror, pull all hair away from your face. Using a bar of soap, draw the outline of your face on the mirror. Stand back. What is your facial shape?
- Gather recent photographs of yourself (full-face) to determine your facial shape.
- Obtain another person's reaction to the question, "What is the shape of my face?"

FACE FLATTERY

One of the first principles cosmeticians learn is this:
Light maximizes and dark minimizes.
Keeping this in mind while working with your makeup will enable you to effect changes that actually alter your appearance by enhancing the good points and playing down the bad ones. Study yourself in the mirror. Stand back and get the overall impression. Now get close to the mirror and analyze each feature from all angles. Get to know your face well so you can work with it properly.

Undertoners

Few people have skin of uniform color. Even without noticeable blotches, freckles, and shadows, there are undertones of shading and color, so the first step in making up after applying your moisturizer is to balance out the skin tone. Foundation accomplishes this purpose to a large extent, but for a really smooth look, check out undertoners. These are liquid colors that neutralize the skin's undertones, complement the surface skin color, and offset any sallowness or ruddiness. Some cosmetic firms have an undertoner that is good for all skin types. We prefer the lotions that come in shades, generally apricot for dark complexions, white for medium complexions, and green for sallow or pale complexions.

Apply lightly with fingertips and smooth over entire face. The key to a successful undertoner is the lightest touch possible.

Concealer

Since most people do have some shadows or bags under the eyes, general use of a concealer is recommended. This is usually a cream in stick form, tube, or in a jar. Some women use their foundation as a concealer, circling the eye with it. Whichever works for you, be certain to match your concealer to the shade closest to the overall color of your complexion, and blot transparent or baby powder over the concealer before applying the rest of your makeup.

Foundation

Tools:
- Makeup sponge
- Powder puff or pad

All complexions benefit from a foundation. On a flawless complexion, a foundation will impart a protective covering from the environment and a smooth base for applying other forms of makeup. If the color of your skin has only a slight uneven tone or texture, foundation is the remedy. Even blemishes can, to an extent, be concealed.

Your skin type and its condition are the two factors involved in selecting the type of foundation you need.

COVERAGE:
    SHEER allows natural skin tone to shine through.
    LIGHT hides tiny lines and discolorations.
    MEDIUM hides light veins and blemishes.
    OPAQUE does not allow any skin color to show through.
    MEDICATED is used by people with acne.

FINISH:
    SHINY
    MOIST
    MATTE

CHOOSING COLOR

Foundation is now available in so many shades that there will be one close to your natural skin color. Darker or lighter shades may exaggerate any imperfections on the face. The easiest method for selecting the right shade is to try it directly on your face. This isn't always possible, so the next best place is the inside of the wrist, as this area most closely resembles the color of facial skin. If after repeated attempts you are unable to find a suitable color, have one professionally blended by a cosmetician. Remember that skin tones change from summer dark to winter pale, so adjust your makeup accordingly.

APPLICATION

Foundation, whether in cream, liquid or gel form, should spread smoothly over the skin. People with dry skin can buy foundation with added moisturizers in an oil base; those with oily skin can purchase it with a water base.

The first step in application is to dot foundation on the forehead, eyelids, nose, cheeks, chin, and neck. Using the fingertips or a damp sponge, follow the facial directionals in the illustration. This is the only exception to the facial directionals given in the skin-care section; using these particular movements for the application of foundation will keep the facial hairs from being pushed in the wrong direction. Gently blend the edges of foundation well into the hairline and under the chin. Start with a thin application; you can always apply more.

Highlighters and Contourers

Remember the basic principle: Light maximizes and dark minimizes. With highlighters and contourers you can make less attractive features recede, achieve facial symmetry, and draw attention to your best beauty assets. Use products specially formulated for this purpose, or use varying shades of foundation. Study your face, deciding which areas should be played up and which should be played down. After applying either highlighter or contourer, be sure to blend the edges discreetly into your foundation.

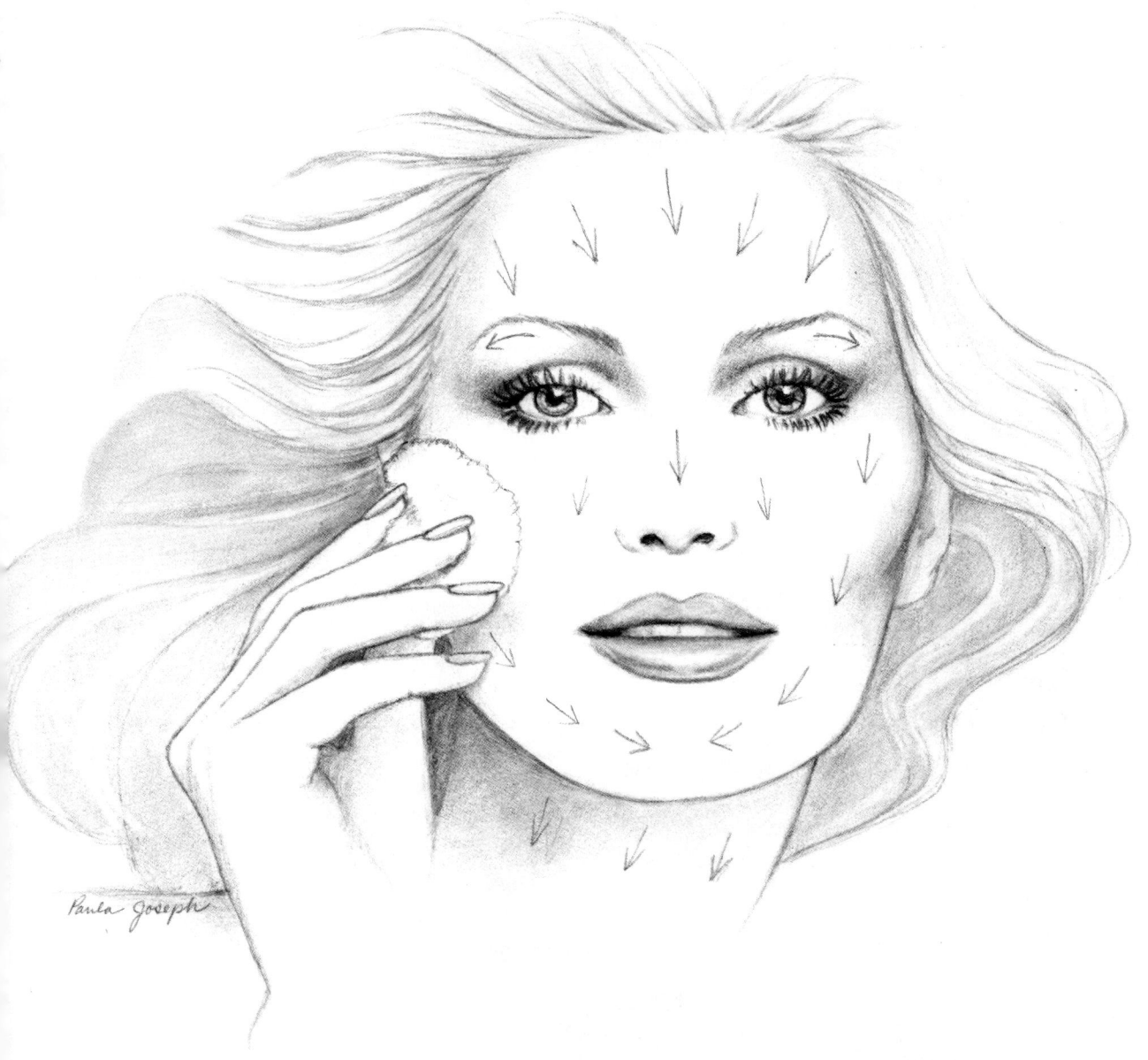

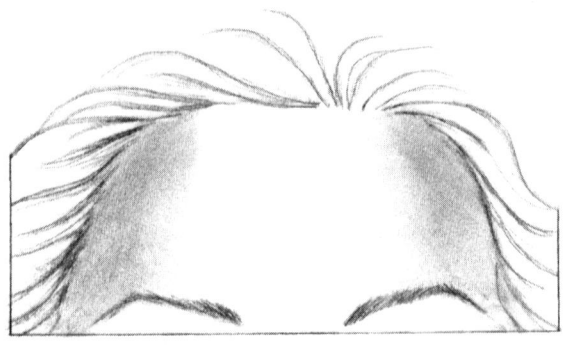

Wide forehead
Contourer

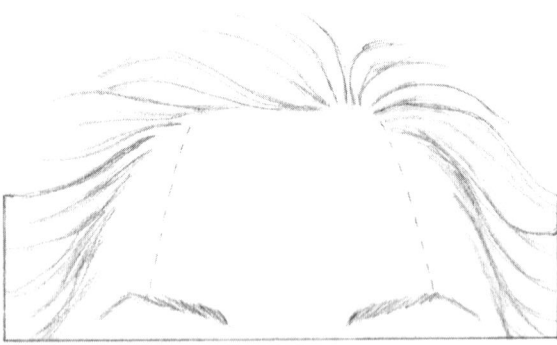

Narrow forehead
Highlighter

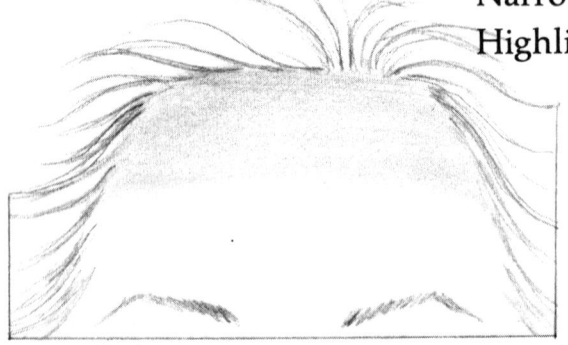

Long forehead
Contourer

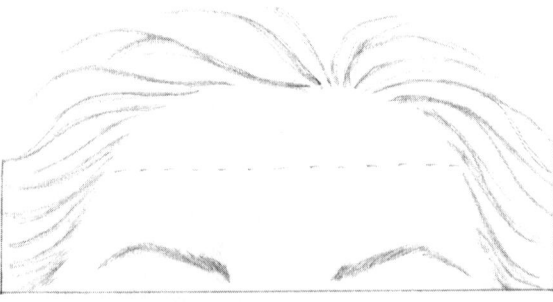

Short forehead
Highlighter

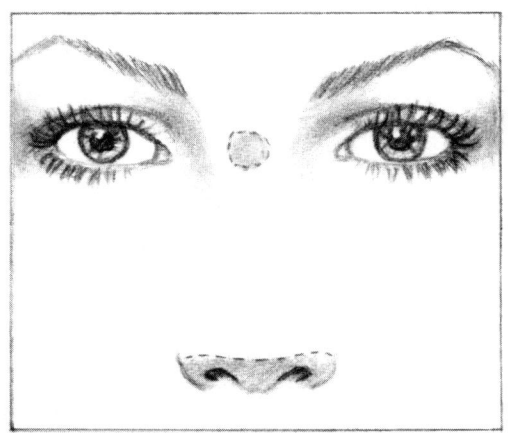

Long nose
Contourer

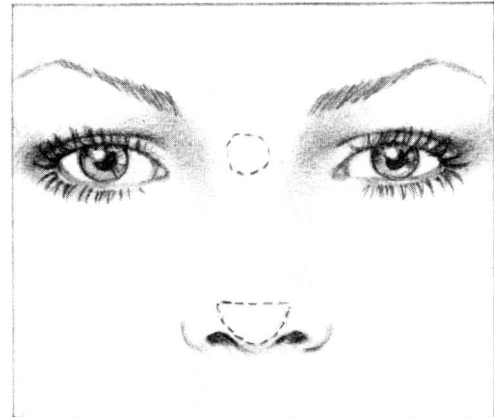

Short nose
Highlighter

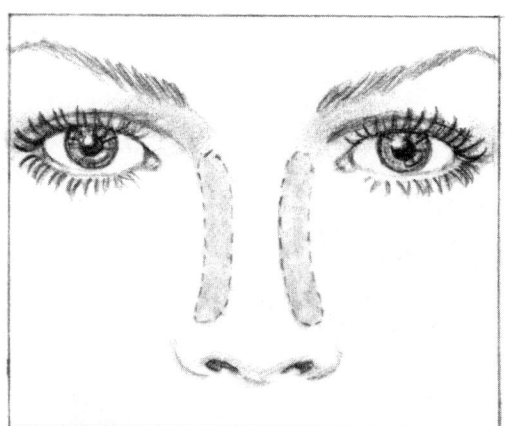

Wide nose

Contourer

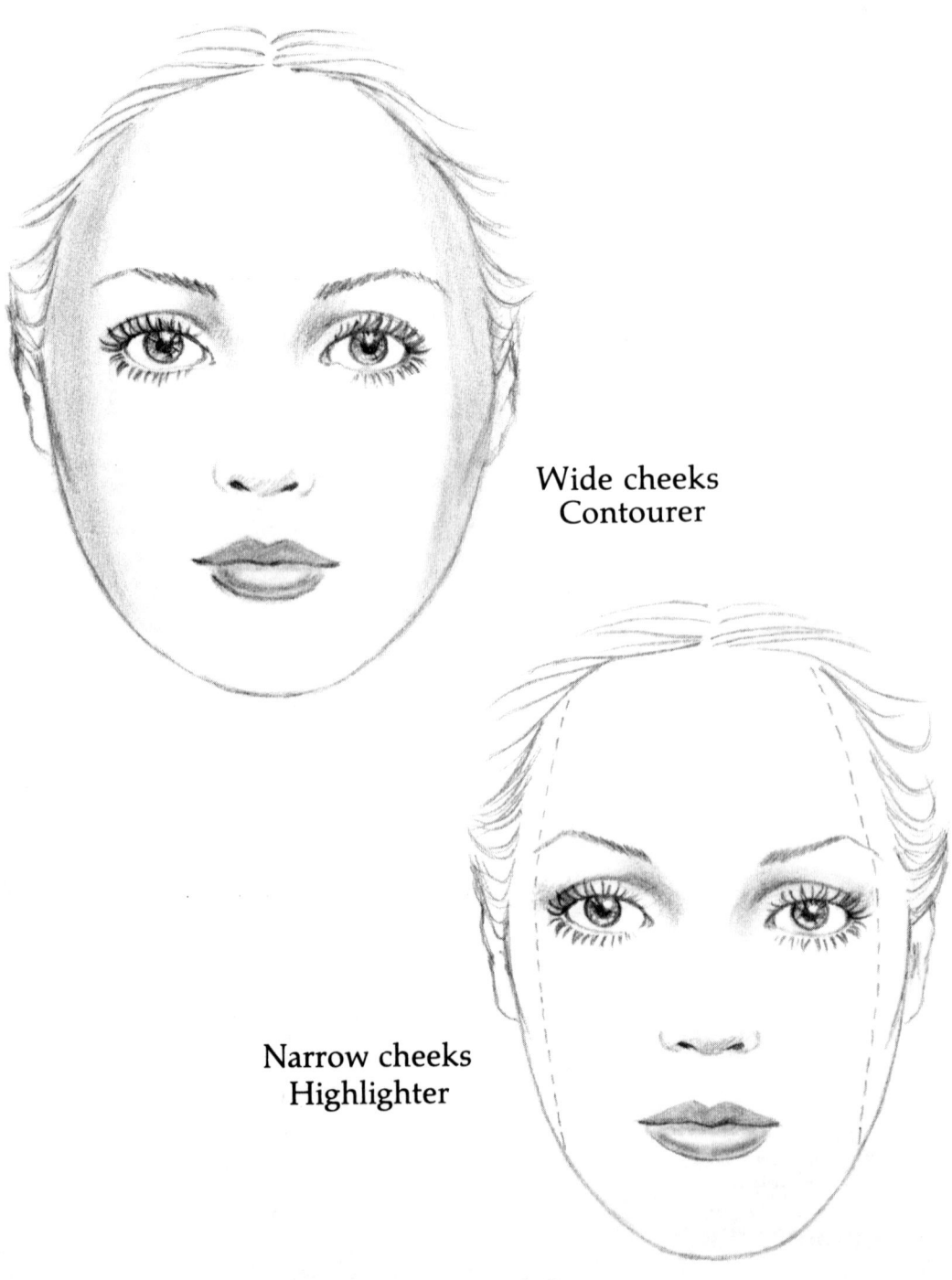

Wide cheeks
Contourer

Narrow cheeks
Highlighter

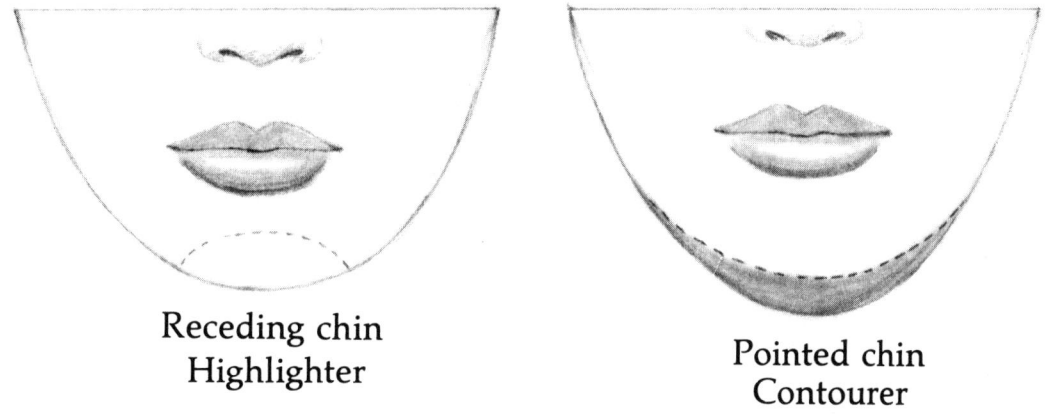

Receding chin
Highlighter

Pointed chin
Contourer

Powder

Powder is used to set makeup, helping it to cling smoothly and evenly, and to offset shine. It comes in either pressed or loose form in a translucent shade. Both forms should be applied with a light touch, concentrated on oily areas such as the nose, the center of the face, the chin, and the forehead. Be especially careful when applying pressed powder not to pull on delicate facial tissues. Powder isn't a makeup necessity; if you like a fresh, shiny look, omit it altogether.

Tips

- If skin is oily, use a makeup sponge, not the fingertips.
- Never rub on foundation; apply it gently.
- Foundation color appears one shade darker in the bottle than it actually is.
- Use loose powder on top of your foundation; pressed powder will smear its application.
- For a shimmering effect, try loose translucent powder with light reflectants added.
- Carry loose or pressed powder with you for quick touch-ups.

Eyes

Eyes are the most individualized feature of our faces, for they are seen in almost as many variations as fingerprints. Different makeup techniques cannot make your eyes look like your favorite model's, but who would want that, as much of the eyes' appeal stems from their uniqueness. Makeup can make your eyes appear large, sparkling, and beautiful.

Tools:

- Makeup sponge
- Eye liner pencils
- Eye shadow brushes

Liners

During the reign of the Cleopatra look in the early 1960s, liners were meant to be noticed. Now they look softer and are smudged gently around the eye in strategic places depending upon eye shape. They still lend a dramatic touch and serve to make lashes appear longer, which is the main purpose of liners. Liquid liner isn't as popular now as pencils, since it's easier to achieve the smudged effect with the latter. The colors most flattering to everyone are shades of brown, with smoky taupes or charcoal grays a close second. Midnight blue is great for nighttime wear. Black, once the great favorite, is too severe and unnatural for today's look. If you have almond-shaped eyes, smudge a thin line of liner along the lid. Circling the entire eye gives a dramatic look. Women with other eye shapes should consult the illustrations on the following pages.

Tips

- Soften pencil liners by running them under hot water.
- Substitute dark shadow in place of liner.

Shadows

Here is where you will put the light-dark principle into the most practice, using colors in many hues and in matte or shiny finishes to make the eyes bigger and brighter. For obvious reasons, women with oily skin are better off with powders, and dry-skinned women do better with creams. Some powders, creams, and pencils contain moisturizers, and may be purchased in waterproof form if long-lasting wear is needed. If your favorite shadow isn't waterproof, apply a clear sealer especially formulated for this purpose. You may apply colors with a brush, sponge, or fingers; just be sure to blend colors into one another and fade out the edges.

There are so many contributing factors regarding color selection that it's primarily a personal choice. Take into account the color of your eyes, hair, skin tones, and clothing. Since eye shadow is worn to accent the eyes' color, it is the most important factor in selecting proper shades, but do use this particular guide loosely.

COLOR GUIDE FOR SHADOW SELECTION

BLUE EYES	GREEN EYES	HAZEL EYES	BROWN EYES	GRAY EYES
Plum	Plum	Muted green and blue	Any color, especially:	Silver
Charcoal	Brown	Muted turquoise	Mauve	Gray
Gray	Muted blue	Plum	Cinnamon	Muted beige
Brown	Muted turquoise	Yellow	Plum	Muted blue
Muted green	Teal		Brown	Soft teal

BLUE EYES	GREEN EYES	HAZEL EYES	BROWN EYES	GRAY EYES
Turquoise	Navy	Brown	Deep green	Taupe
Mauve	Gold	Gold	Burgundy	
Teal	Copper	Copper	Taupe	

SHADING

A popular style for shading has been to color the eyelid, deepen the crease between the lid and brow with a dark contour shade, and highlight the area beneath the brow with a light shade or highlighter. There are other techniques of shading, and the chart on eye shapes will explain them. Those of you with almond-shaped eyes may want to try some of these for a different look.

Eye Shapes

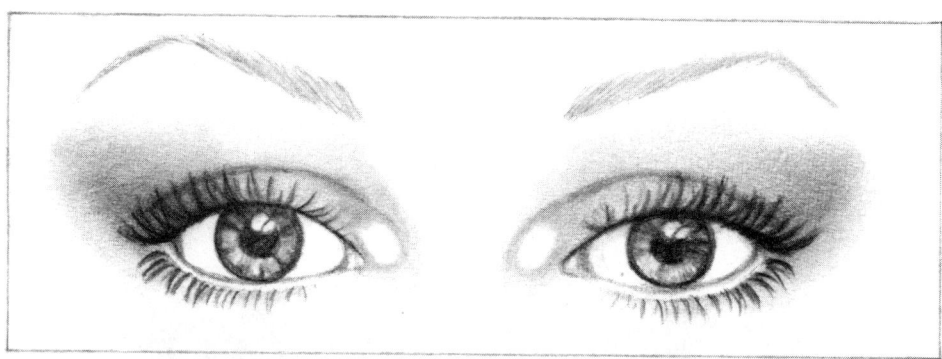

CLOSE-SET EYES

1. Use light-colored shadow on inner half of upper lid, medium shade on outer half, and blend.
2. Extend color out from eyelid toward hairline.
3. Dot highlighter in inner corner of eye.
4. Extend liner a touch beyond outer edge.
5. Apply an extra coat of mascara on outer lashes.
6. Pluck inner end of brows so that they appear further apart, keeping them light and thin.

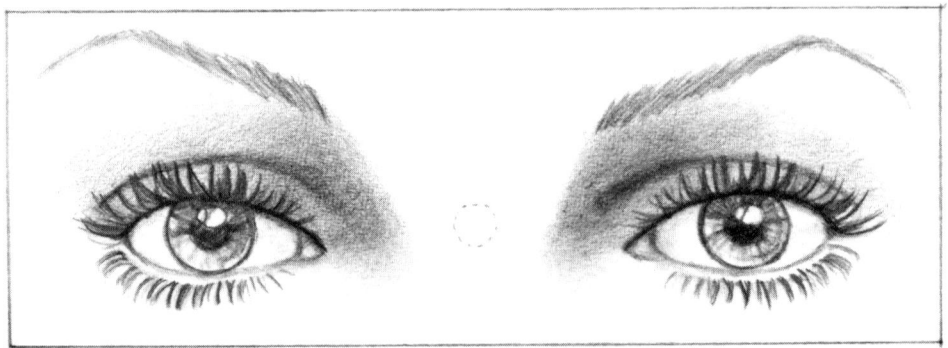

WIDE-SET EYES

1. Start shadow closer to nose, using a dark shadow on inner half of upper lid, medium shade on outer half, and blend.
2. Dot highlighter on bridge of nose.
3. Extend liner all the way to the inner corner of eye.
4. Concentrate mascara in center of eye.

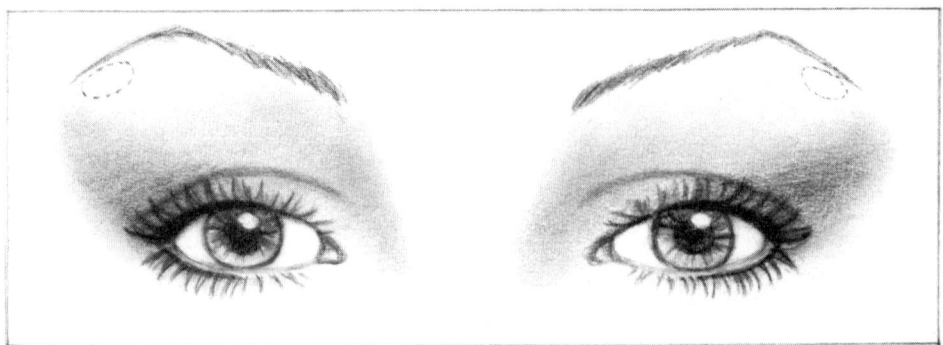

SMALL EYES

1. Use light-colored shadow on inner half of eye from lashes to brow, dark shadow on outer half of eye from lashes to brow, extending beyond outer edges.
2. Dot highlighter right under outer edge of brow.
3. Keep liner on outer half of eye.
4. Keep eyebrows light and thin.

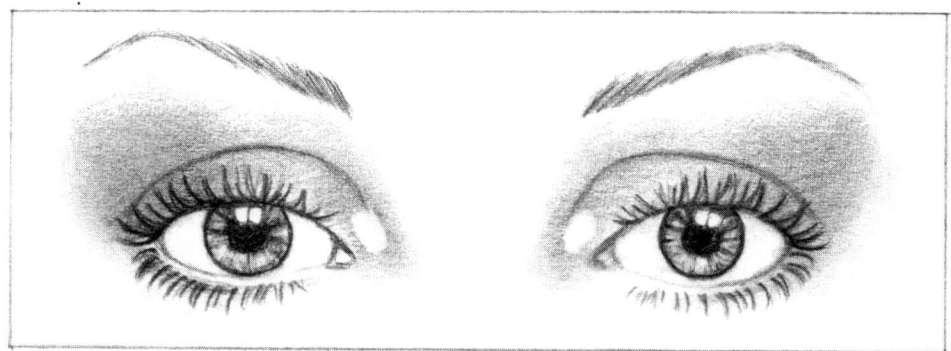

DEEP-SET EYES

1. Use light-colored shadow on inner half of upper lid, darker shadow on outer half of upper lid.
2. Do not darken crease of eye.
3. Dot highlighter in inner corners.
4. Do not use liner.

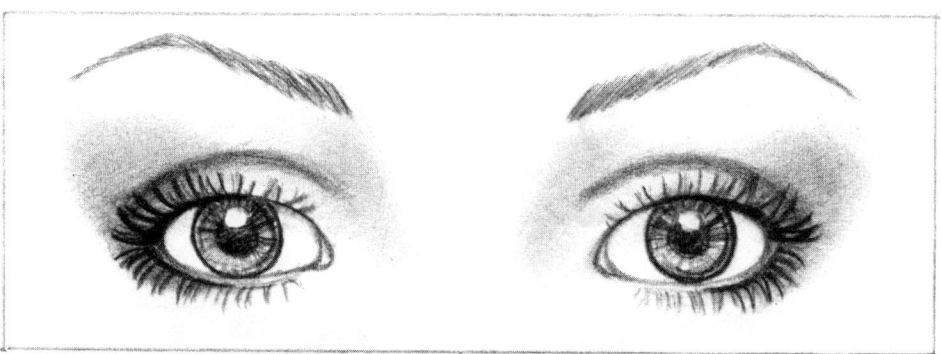

ROUND EYES

1. Use medium shadow across outer half of lid and under lower lashes at outside corner.
2. Use dark shadow in crease.
3. Line only outer half of eye.
4. Add mascara to outer lashes.

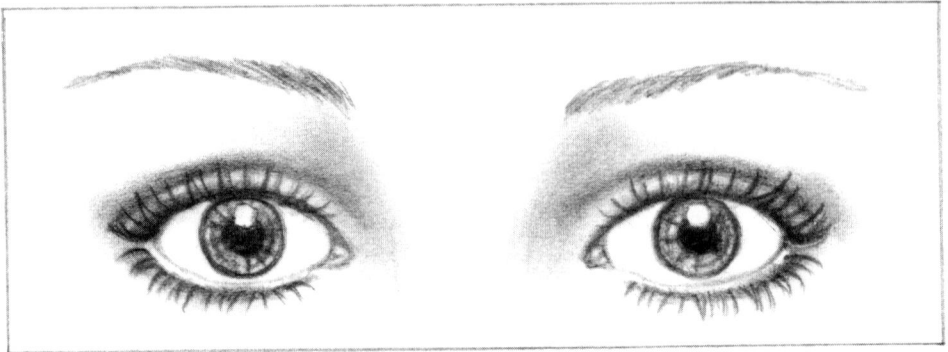

BULGING OR PUFFY EYES

1. Avoid light or shiny shadows.
2. Use a highlighter in inner corners.
3. Use a dark shadow in crease of eye.
4. Smudge liner from inner corner to outer edge on upper and lower lids.
5. Keep brows in a straight line.

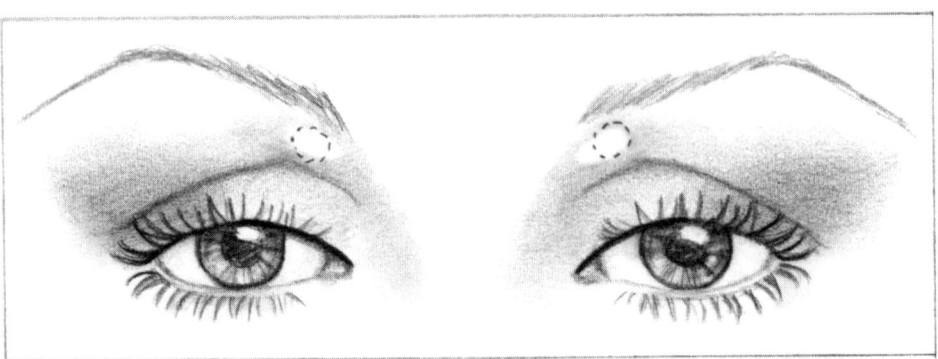

DROOPY LIDS

1. Use a light shadow along inner half of upper lid, dark shadow along outer half.
2. Use dark matte shadow where lid begins to droop.
3. Dot highlighter under inner edge of brow.
4. Line from inner top edge to pupil.
5. With pencil, extend brows slightly on outer edges.

Mascara

Tools:
- Mascara
- Curler
- Eyebrow brush-comb

Mascara is the one essential step in your eye makeup. Each eyelash is like a small exclamation point accenting your eye, and mascara dramatizes this effect. No other item, not even lipstick, can add glamour to a face as easily as the ingredient found in those little wands. Important, yes; difficult, no. In fact, mascara is the easiest of all to master. First, select the type and brand of mascara you like in the proper shade. There are powder and cake mascaras, but we recommend those that come in the wand form with applicator. Some formulas have added conditioners (a great idea) or lash lengtheners. Some are waterproof. Experiment to learn which is the best for you.

Proper shade is determined by hair color.

HAIR COLOR	MASCARA
Black	Black
Brunette	Black
Brown	Black or dark brown
Light brown	Dark brown; tip lashes with black
Dark blond	Dark blond; tip lashes with black
Light blond	Brown; tip lashes with dark brown
Gray	Charcoal gray; tip lashes with black

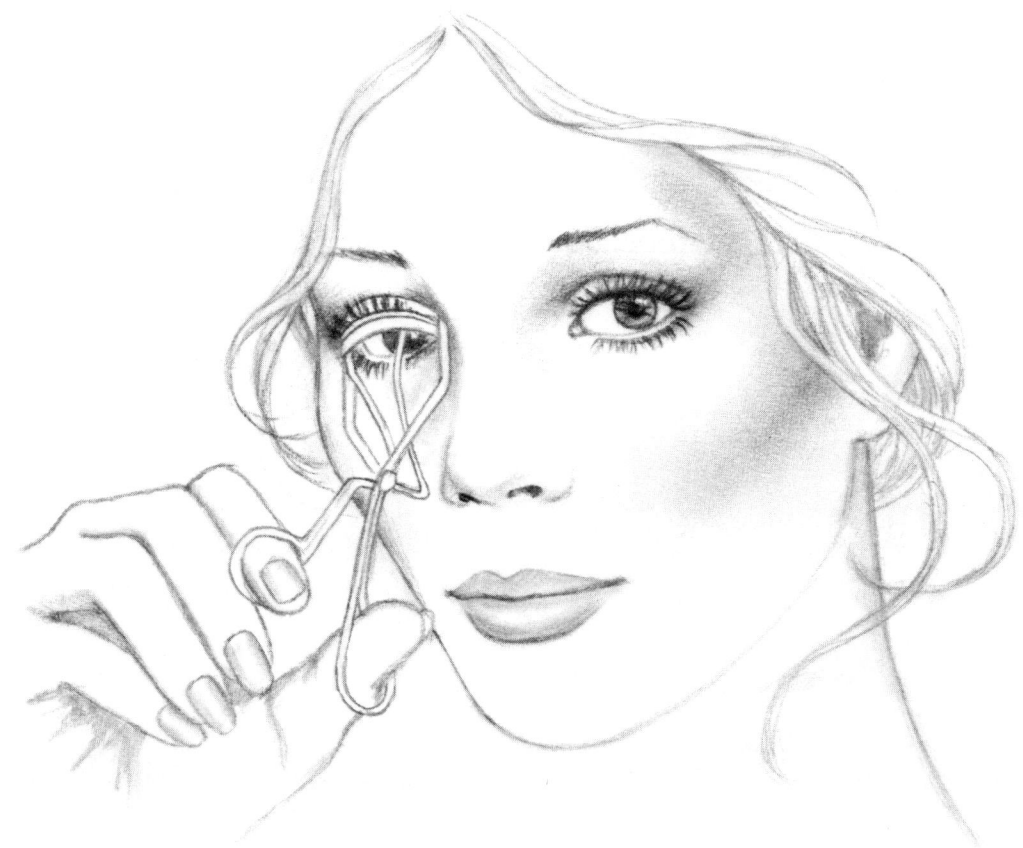

    Curl your lashes when all eye makeup is in place except for mascara. An eyelash curler is very simple to use and will not pull out lashes as long as you keep the rubber pad clean and unworn; remember to open the curler fully before removing from eyelashes (sounds silly, but people have forgotten, to their dismay), and never curl lashes once mascara has been applied. All it takes is a 10-second hold, and your lashes will turn up.

Now apply one thin coat of mascara from base of upper lashes to the tips and from base of lower lashes to the tips. Reinsert wand in tube, and allow time for lashes to dry thoroughly. Comb lashes apart with an eyebrow comb-brush. Reapply mascara, powdering the lashes beforehand if you desire extra thickness. Comb again when dry. Check to make certain that lashes are of equal intensity.

TO AVOID SMEARING

Use waterproof mascara.

●

Hold a tissue beneath lower lashes while applying mascara.

●

Use a sealer.

FOR A SPECIAL LOOK

Use a third coat of mascara on tips of lashes and/or outer lashes for a wide-eyed look.

●

Use midnight blue shade at night.

●

Coat the upper side of lashes before coating the underside.

One final word: Please discard mascara, whether it is used up or not, after four months, because the dark, moist environment is a perfect breeding place for bacteria.

False Lashes

Tools:
- False lashes
- Adhesive

Since modern mascaras have become so rich, women do not have to wear false lashes on a daily basis. For certain occasions, however, they do add a special look. You don't want this makeup aid to be noticed; rather, the object of false lashes is to make your own lashes look thicker and thereby enhance the eye. Therefore, purchase a pair of lashes that most closely match your own in color, trim them to a length not any longer than your own (vary the length of individual lashes, as your own lashes vary in length), and never extend them beyond the natural line on either side of the eye.

To apply: Spread a thin line of adhesive (surgical adhesive works well) on the base of the false lash. Press it gently into position as close to your own lash as possible. If the false lashes don't look right or feel secure, take them off and repeat the procedure. To remove, grip the outer corner of the false lash strip and firmly pull across; it should come off easily. If not, try applying some baby oil to the base, then pull. To clean your lashes, let them soak for five minutes in alcohol and dry on a tissue; don't use them again for at least an hour. Or soak them in a solution of water and detergent for half an hour, and gently rinse them off completely.

Eyebrows

Tools:
- Tweezers
- Alcohol
- Eyebrow brush-comb
- Manicure scissors
- Eyebrow pencil or powder

Beautiful eyebrows are rarely remarked upon, primarily because they focus attention onto the eyes rather than themselves. Ugly, shapeless brows, however, can be the most noticed feature on a face, leaving the onlooker with a negative impression of your appearance or an incorrect idea of your attitude. As people speak, focus on their eyebrows and you'll soon see how important this small feature is.

Proper brow-shaping and maintenance are two of the least difficult steps involved in a beauty regimen. The basic rule is to follow the natural line, for the most flattering shape is determined by each individual's face. Most brows follow the bone line that protrudes above the eye; remove hairs that grow below this bone. To refine your natural shape, stand in front of a mirror with a pencil in hand and:

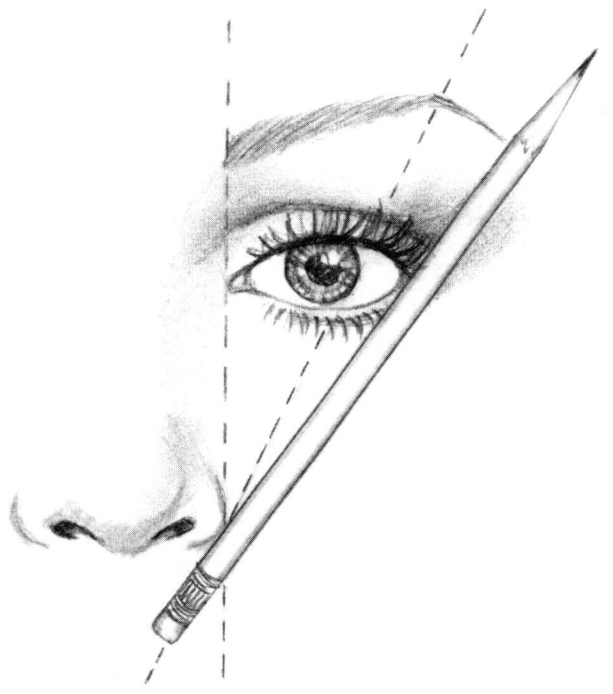

1. Hold pencil vertically against each side of the nose, point nearest brow and eraser nearest nostril. Tweeze any hairs that extend beyond pencil over the nose.
2. Keeping the point of the pencil in place, move the top end diagonally to a point right above the outside edge of the iris of your eye. This is where the brow should arch. Tweeze stray hairs that are beneath the arch or tend to obscure it, taking care not to make brow too thin.
3. Move the pencil to the outside of your eye, and tweeze brows that extend beyond the point where the pencil meets the brow.

4. Keep the area between brows tweezed to avoid an untamed look.

5. Strive for a smooth line, with the brow the same width over each eye across to the arch at which point it tapers delicately to the end.

TWEEZING

Don't be reluctant to pluck. It isn't painful when done correctly.

1. Clean tips of tweezers with alcohol.
2. Brush brows up and back in place.
3. Wipe brow area with astringent or toner.
4. Tweeze quickly, in direction of hair growth, one hair at a time.
5. Apply astringent afterward to avoid infection and wash tweezers.

Brows that are still too thick can be trimmed with manicure scissors. Brush the brow straight up, and carefully trim the edges that exceed the brow line. Trim just a few hairs at a time; you can always trim more away later.

EYEBROW COLOR

Correct color is determined by hair color. Dark-haired women should keep their brows one or two shades lighter than their hair, and light-haired women should keep their brows one or two shades darker than their hair. If your brows are light, pencil or powder applied in short, feathery strokes will rectify that. If your brows are too dark, cover them with foundation or highlighter, and then apply the correct shade of pencil or powder. It is possible to have brows bleached or dyed, a very dangerous process that should never be attempted at home. Dyes and bleaches have chemicals in them that can cause blindness.

Tips
- Keep after stray hairs daily
- If you find tweezing painful, numb the area with ice or open the pores with heat.
- Buy a tweezer with pointed tips for fine hairs.

- For those having difficulty determining proper brow shape, get a professional tweeze and thereafter follow that line.
- Brush brows daily.
- Control bushy or wild brows with a dab of petroleum jelly.

Cheek Color

Tools:
- Brush
- Sponge
- Color

Cheek color softens the angles of the face and provides skin with a healthy glow. It's available in stick, powder, cream, or gel form. The stick is applied directly. Powder forms have brush applicators. Creams and gels are applied with damp sponges or fingertips.

Cheek color should harmonize with your foundation, your lipstick color, and your wardrobe. Use the chart of suggested cheek colors as a guideline.

SUGGESTED CHEEK COLORS

	PINK or RUDDY TONE	YELLOW or SALLOW	OLIVE	PALE
LIGHT SKIN SHADE	Brick ● Red	Peach ● Pink ● Amber	Deep peach ● Red	Light pink ● Coral
MEDIUM	Brick ● Red	Peach ● Amber ● Bronze ● Pink	Deep peach ● Red	Pink ● Coral

DARK	Brick	Peach	Rose	Dark pink
	●	●		●
	Red	Amber		Coral
		●		
		Bronze		
BLACK	Brick	Amber		Deep russet
	●	●		●
	Red	Cinnamon		Burgundy
	●			
	Mulberry			

Skin with a *tawny* tone, no matter how light or dark, will show off any cheek color attractively.

Cheek color can enhance or diminish facial features, so it's important to understand where to apply i. Determining your correct facial shape will help.

1. Study your face in the mirror, and find your cheekbones. Feel to see where they start at the top and bottom and how they continue away from the nose.
2. Pucker your lips, and apply either a darker foundation or a darker cheek color in this hollow, following upward to the end of the cheekbone.

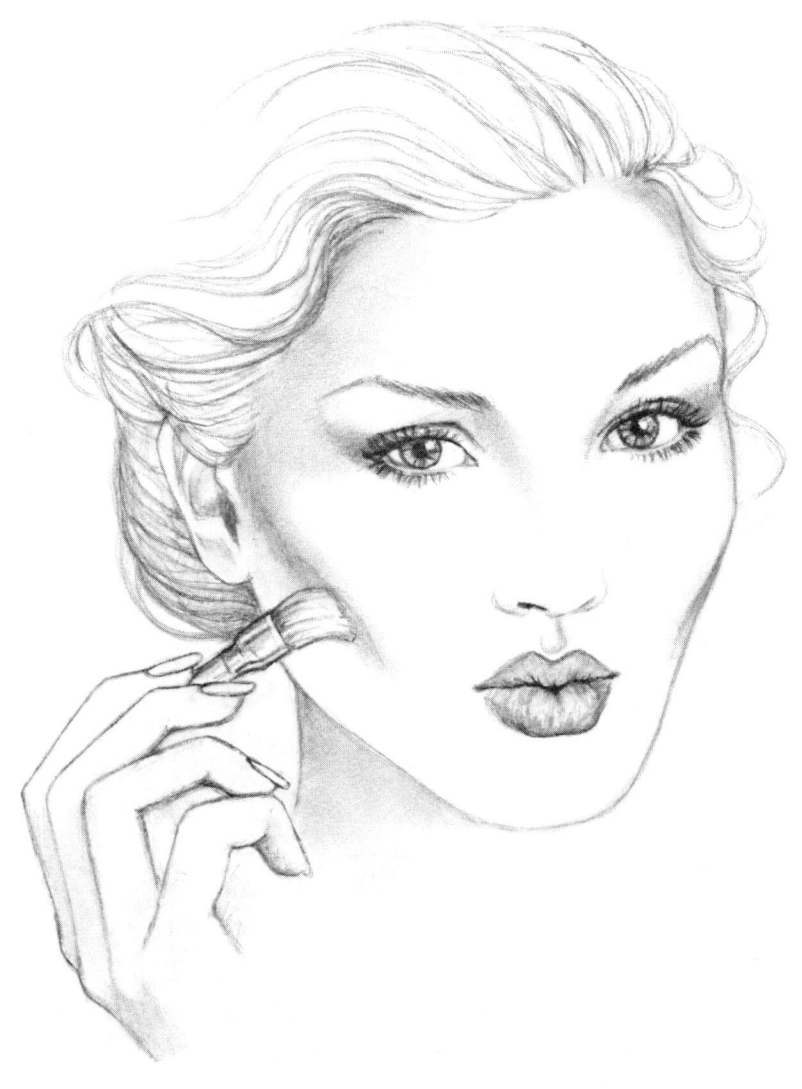

3. Now apply your cheek color to the fullest part of the cheeks, starting from directly below the pupil of the eye out to the end of the cheekbone.

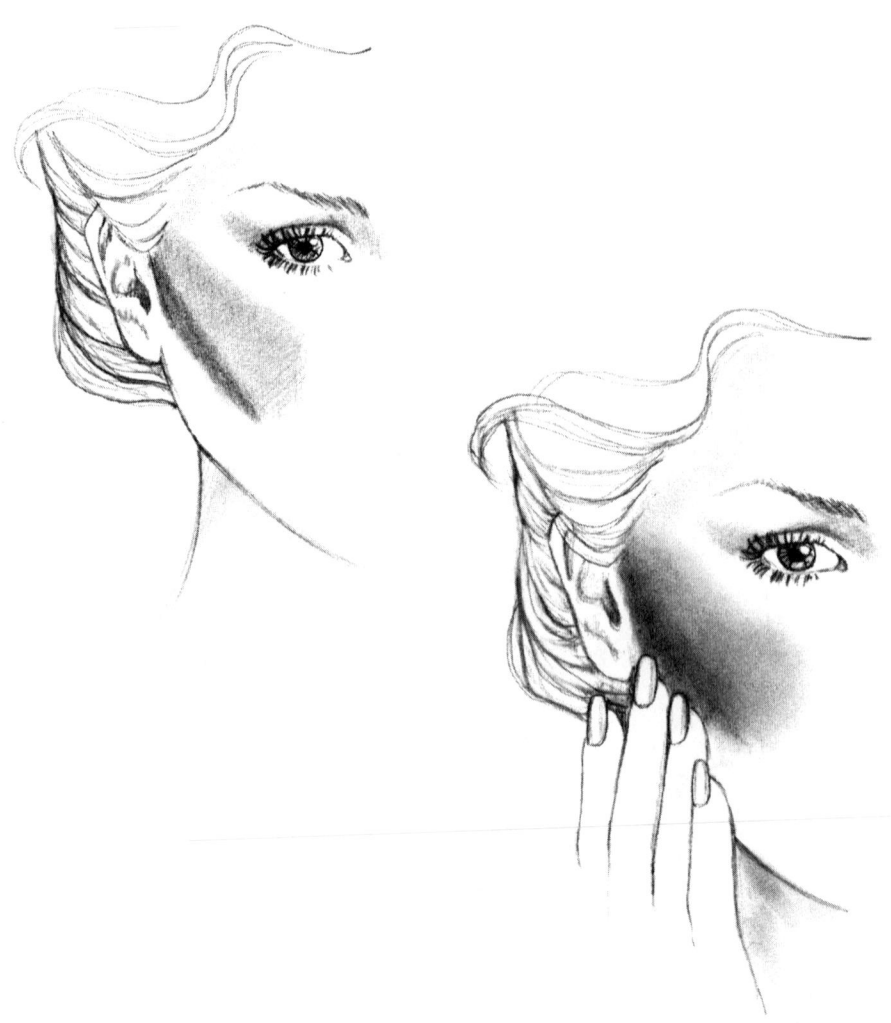

4. Blend the edges of the contouring and the cheek color together to avoid looking artificial.

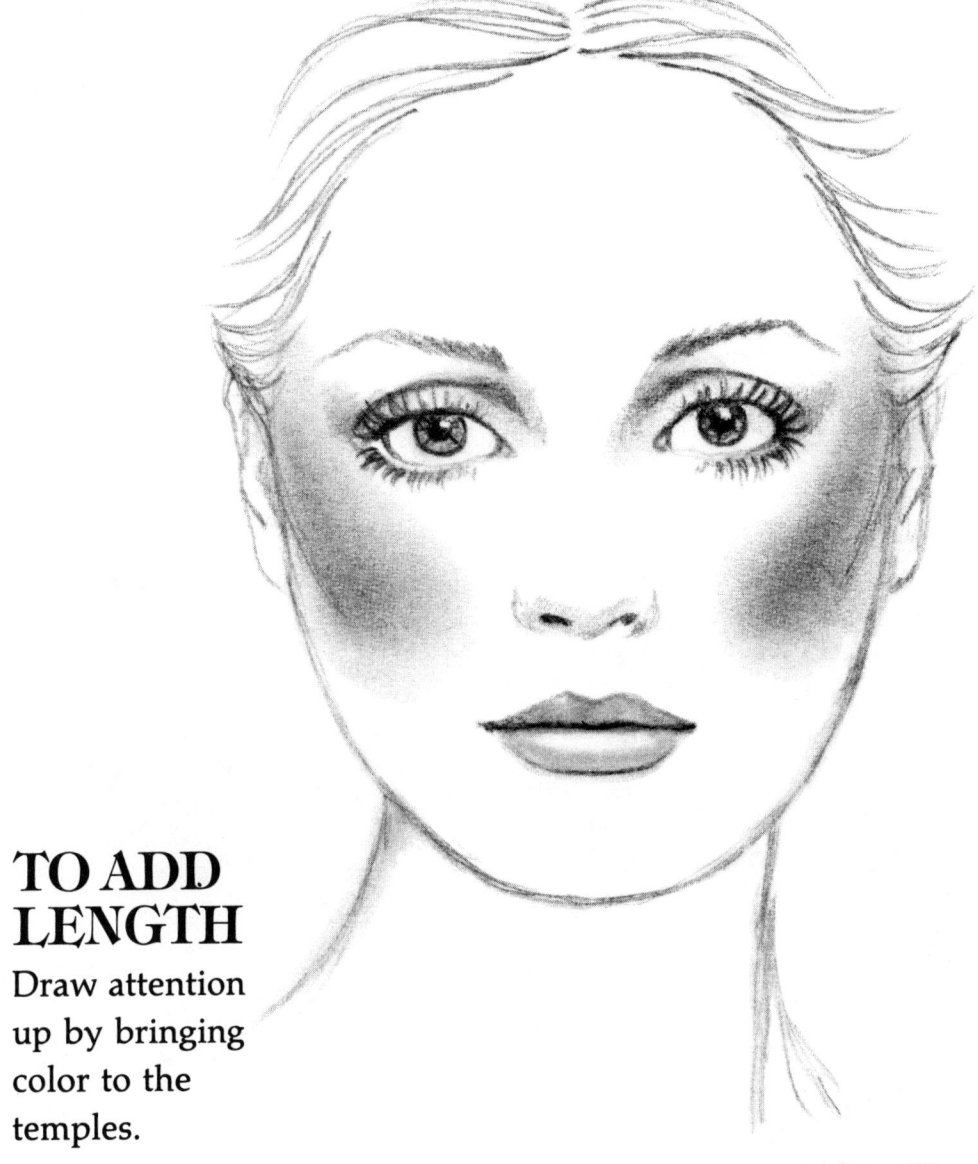

TO ADD LENGTH

Draw attention up by bringing color to the temples.

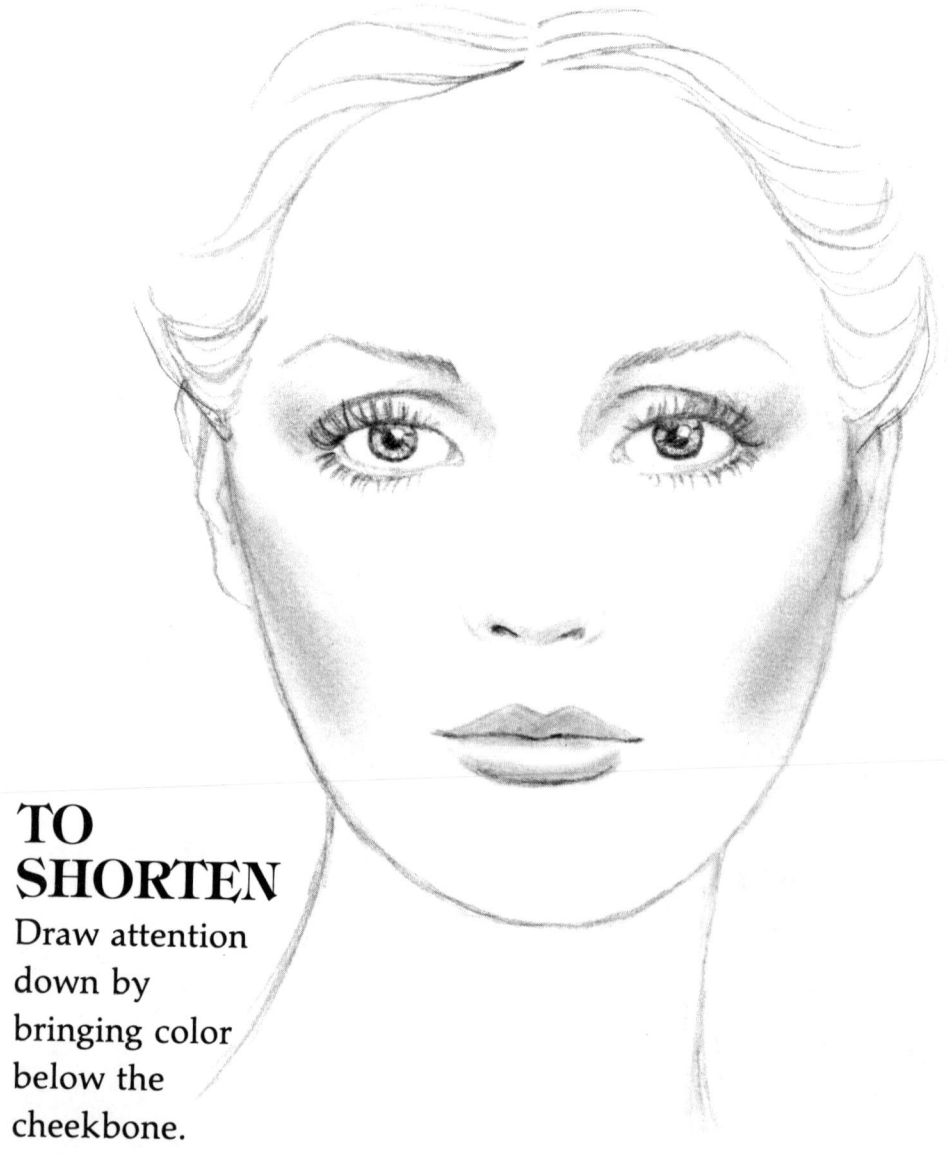

TO SHORTEN

Draw attention down by bringing color below the cheekbone.

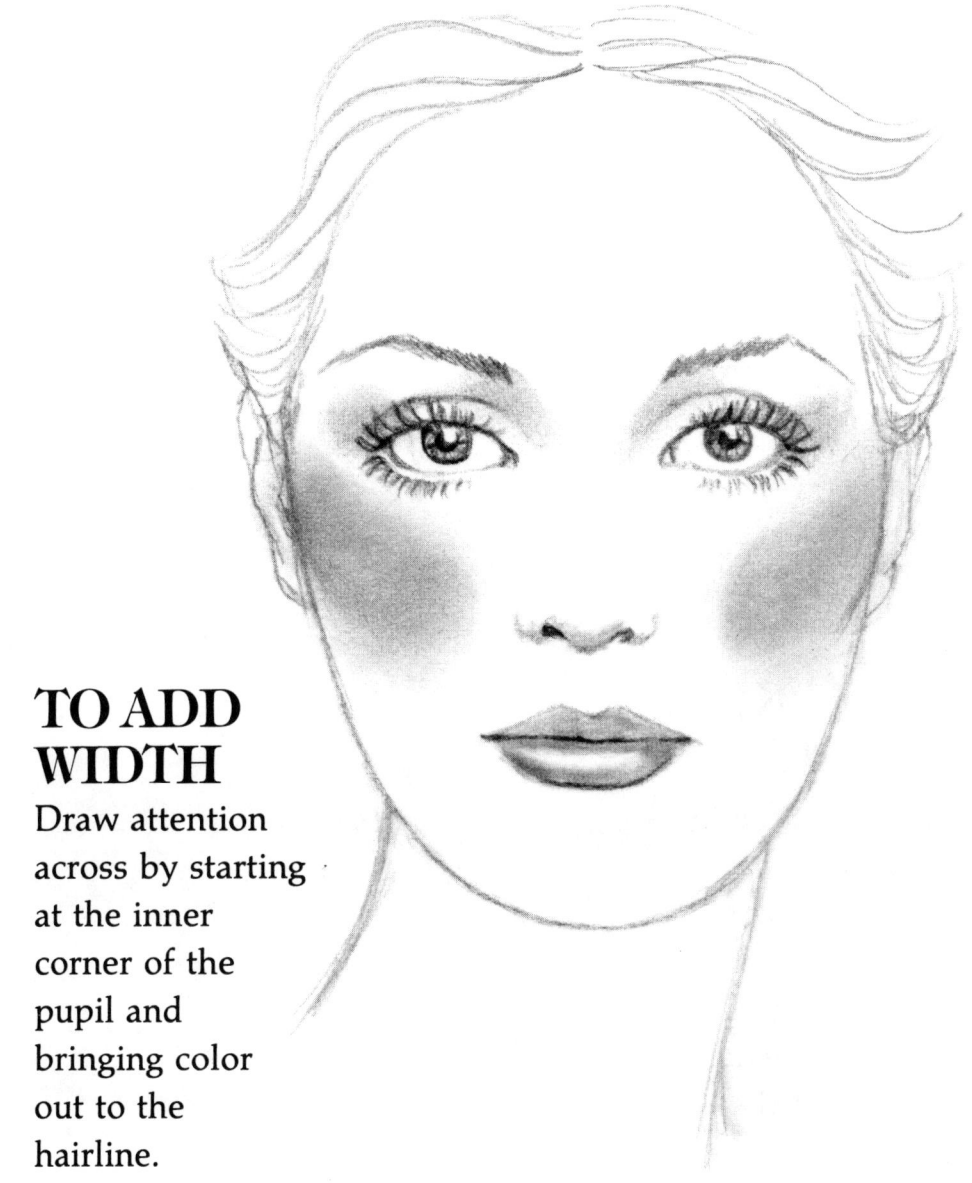

TO ADD WIDTH
Draw attention across by starting at the inner corner of the pupil and bringing color out to the hairline.

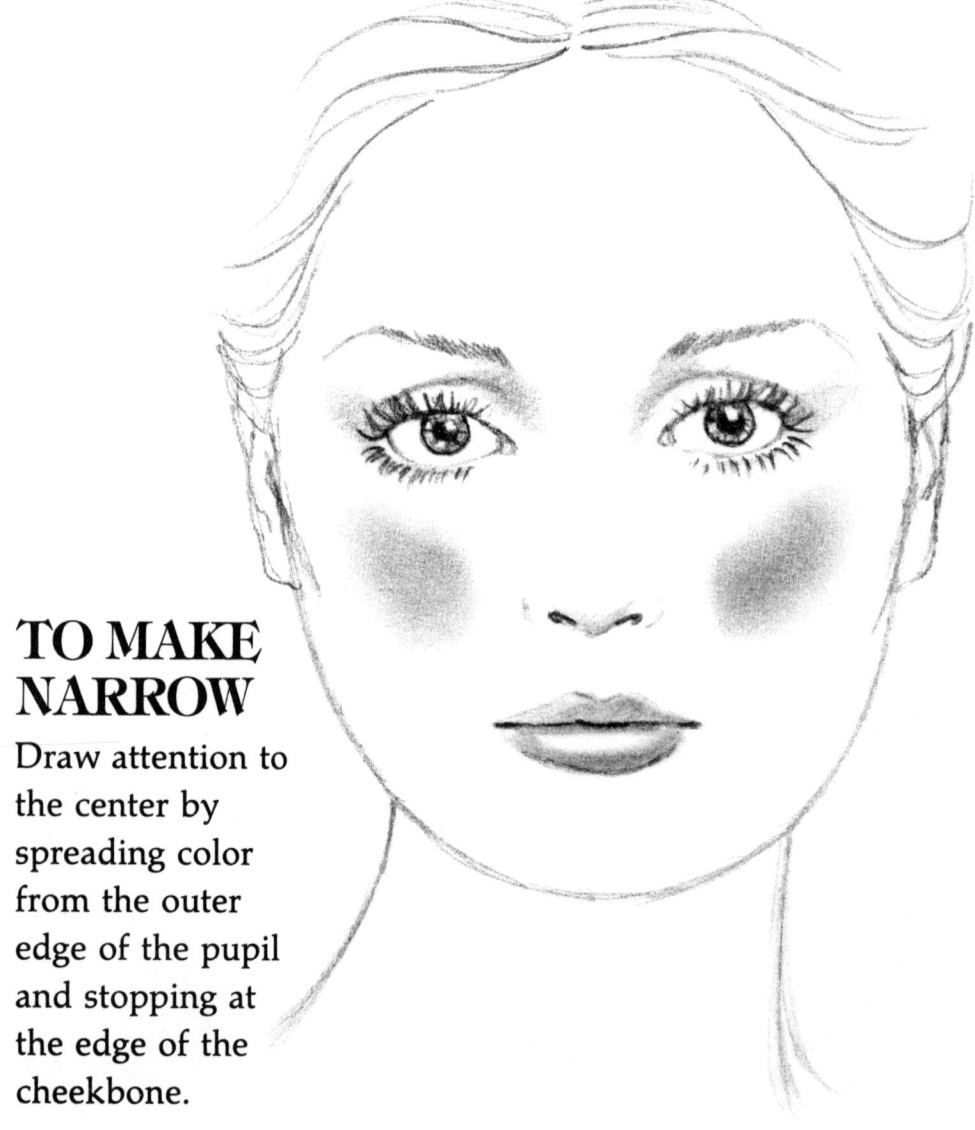

TO MAKE NARROW

Draw attention to the center by spreading color from the outer edge of the pupil and stopping at the edge of the cheekbone.

Tips
- Apply cheek color down the sides of the neck for the appearance of a longer neck. Blend well.
- Use a dab of cheek color on the chin to highlight.
- Use only a dash of color on tanned skin.
- Cheek color belongs on cheeks. It should not be too close to eyes or nose.

Lips

Tools:
- Lip brush
- Lip pencil

TYPES OF LIPSTICK

The type of lipstick to use is up to the individual. Those with conditioners or moisturizers are superior to those without them, as the additional ingredients protect delicate skin.

CREAM LIPSTICKS contain color without shine.

FROST LIPSTICKS contain color with an iridescent glow. Don't equate shine with moisturizer; check to be certain moisturizer has been added.

GLOSSES have a clear, shiny base, and are usually worn over a cream lipstick to provide the mouth with extra protection and more gleam. They may also be worn alone.

LASTING-COLOR LIPSTICKS are basic colors that have been formulated to last for long periods of time.

TRANSLUCENT LIPSTICKS add just a hint of color.

LIP COLOR

Lip color should harmonize with your foundation shade, cheek color, and the clothes you are wearing. Also read the tips below to aid you in selection of color.

Tips

- To play down large lips, try a shade close to your natural lip color.
- To make small lips appear larger, try a bright, shiny color.
- Avoid frosts if your lips are full.
- Avoid dark shades if your lips are small.
- Avoid shades of orange if your teeth seem yellowed.
- Whenever possible, try shade on before purchasing.

APPLICATION OF COLOR

Definitive shaping of the mouth is dependent upon a clear outline. This sharp edge of color is easier to obtain by using either a lip brush or lip pencil. A lip brush may be purchased at nominal cost and is considered indispensable by most cosmeticians. The brush can be made from natural or manmade bristles. The handle should be at least two to three inches long for better control. Lip pencils resemble eyebrow pencils in form, but the lead is creamier and the shades are in reds and browns. The pencil must be kept sharp.

1. Coat the lip brush with lipstick.
2. Outline the lower lip.
3. Fill in the remaining area of the lower lip with lipstick applied directly from the tube.
4. Outline the upper lip in two steps. Start from the corner of the mouth and draw to the center, then repeat for the other side.
5. Fill in the remaining area of the upper lip with lipstick applied directly from the tube.
6. Wipe excess lipstick off brush.

LIP SHADES

The most perfect lips are of equal depth and equal width, but if these characteristics don't describe your lips, don't despair. With a little practice and the help of a few makeup tricks, your lips can take on a new shape.

AVERAGE

Lucky you! Outline the lips with either a lip brush or lip pencil, and fill in with lipstick.

FULL

Cover edges of the lips with your foundation, and blot with powder; redefine the lips just *inside* the natural lipline with a lip brush or lip pencil, and fill in with lipstick.

THIN

Cover edges of the lips with your foundation, and blot with powder; redefine the lips just outside the natural lipline with a lip brush or lip pencil, and fill in with lipstick.

UPPER LIP TOO FULL LOWER LIP TOO FULL

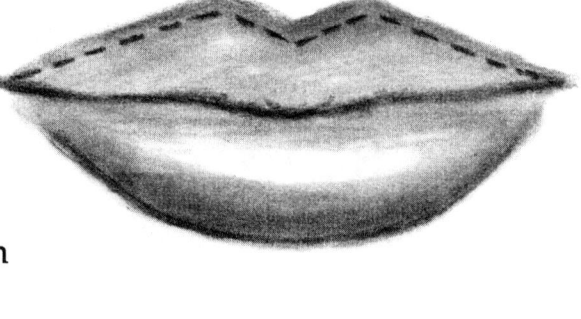

Cover the larger lip with foundation, and blot with powder; redefine the larger lip just inside the natural lipline with a lip brush or lip pencil, and fill in with lipstick. Follow the natural outline of the other lip with a lip brush or pencil, and fill in with lipstick.

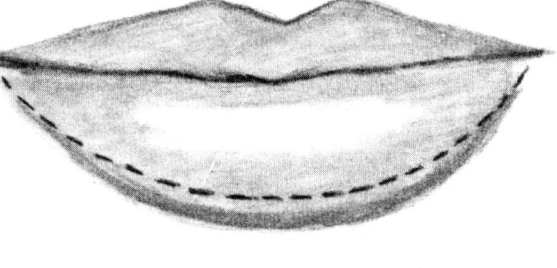

CROOKED UPPER LIP

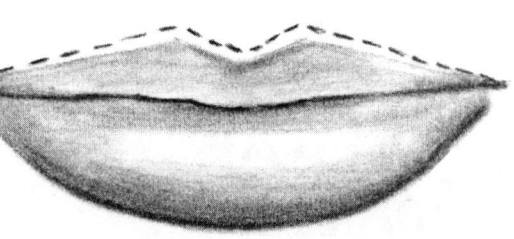

Cover the upper lip with foundation, and blot with powder; straighten the lipline with a pencil or brush just outside the natural lipline. Outline the natural lower lipline, and proceed with lipstick.

UPPER LIP TOO THIN LOWER LIP TOO THIN

Cover the smaller lip with foundation, and blot with powder; redefine the lower lip just outside the natural lipline with a lip brush or pencil, and fill in with lipstick. Follow the natural outline of the other lip with a lip brush or pencil, and fill in with lipstic.

DROOPY CENTER OF UPPER LIP

Apply a vertical white line of light foundation or highlighter through the center of the droop; outline and fill in lips with lipstick.

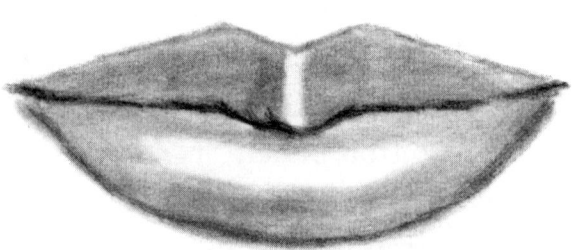

Tips

- To prolong the color of your lipstick, blot an ice-cube to your lips.
- Let lipstick warm up in the sun if it doesn't glide on smoothly.
- Lipstick should look moist and appealing, not caked or layered.
- If teeth have a grayish cast to them, avoid lipsticks with tints of blue.
- To mend a broken lipstick, heat the ends over a low flame and press edges together gently. Let stand for 24 hours.
- Remember, a smile can alter any lips into a pleasing shape.

HIGHLIGHT ON HAIR

Tools: (choose from the following):
- Blow dryer
- Clips
- Comb
- Hairbrush
- Conditioners

- Cream rinse
- Crimping iron
- Curling iron
- Electric rollers
- Hairpins
- Afro pick

The care a woman devotes to her hair is vital to the image she is trying to create. Today's woman wants a no-muss, no-fuss style that can be washed, rinsed, and dried with a minimum of effort for a maximum of effect. This section will serve as an aid in attaining that style and in the maintenance of healthy hair.

The hair, unlike the skin, has no power of self-repair; once the hair shaft becomes damaged it must be cut off. Most hair needs trimming every six weeks or so to keep the ends from straggling. You can avoid some damage, however, by a careful program of cleaning and conditioning.

Select your type of hair from the following lists to determine the methods and products designed for you.

Hair Type

NORMAL HAIR

Shines, retains body from washing to washing.

●

Requires shampooing every three to four days.

- No dandruff.

- Skin type is normal.

OILY HAIR

- Lacks body.

- Requires shampooing every day or so.

- Looks and feels greasy a day after shampooing.

- Hair texture is usually fine.

- Skin type is oily.

DRY HAIR

- Is dull.

Has dandruff.

●

Requires shampooing only once a week.

●

Has static electricity.

●

Skin type is dry.

Care of Hair

After you have identified your personal hair characteristics, the cleaning and conditioning of hair are your next considerations. Check the chart for the type of shampoo and conditioner that you need and the frequency of their use.

HAIR TYPE	TYPE OF SHAMPOO	TYPE OF CONDITIONER
Normal	Use a shampoo specially formulated for normal hair. ● Shampoo every three to four days.	Use a cream rinse to avoid tangles. ● Try a penetrating conditioner once a month. ● Instant conditioner may be used if desired.

Oily	Use a shampoo specially formulated for oily hair. ● Alternate with a gentle shampoo to prevent ends from being damaged. ● Shampoo every day if necessary.	Avoid cream rinses; they attract dirt, which clings to oil. ● Try a penetrating conditioner once a month on ends if they become dry. ● If ends are constantly dry, use instant conditioner after each shampoo on ends.
Dry	Use a shampoo specially formulated for dry hair. ● Shampoo once a week.	Instant conditioners may be used with every washing. ● Try a penetrating conditioner once a month.

Shampoo

Shampooing is the most basic step in caring for the hair. Use the following guidelines to make your hair shine.

1. Massage hair with fingertips before shampooing to loosen and remove excess dirt.
2. Brush out snarls and tangles.
3. Pour a small amount of shampoo into hand, and work a lather; apply the lather directly onto wet hair.
4. Work lather from scalp to ends, and massage scalp with fingertips. Be careful not to scratch the scalp.
5. Rinse with cool water, then rinse again and again, as shampoo left on the hair may cause dulling.
6. Apply conditioner, if required, following the manufacturer's directions.
7. Towel-dry gently to avoid breakage.
8. Remove snarls and tangles with wide-tooth comb.

Going to a Hairdresser

Choosing the right hairdresser can be as important to your beauty image as choosing a doctor is to your physical well-being. A good style cannot be obtained without a good cut. Finding a good hairdresser may take time and effort, but the rewards are well worth it.

Tips

- Listen closely to what other women are saying about their hairdressers; you may be rewarded with some useful information.
- Ask a person whose hair you admire where she has it done and by whom.
- Visit the salon prior to your appointment to view the professional at work.
- Try to determine if the hairdresser is actually listening to you or just doing what he/she prefers.
- Be realistic. First determine if a model has your facial shape, features, and hair characteristics before bringing in a picture of a desired hairstyle.

Choosing a Hairstyle

On the chart below, you will find one or more of your features. To obtain the best overall shape for your hairstyle, incorporate the components for each prominent feature.

FACIAL CHARACTERISTICS		TYPE OF STYLE
Forehead	Wide	Softness and height at crown ● Side part
	Short	Softness and height at crown ● Hair away from forehead

	Long	Wide bangs
		●
		Width and softness at side
	Narrow	Wide bangs
		●
		Side part
Cheekbones	Wide	Softness and height at crown
		●
	Narrow	Straight bangs
		●
		Width and softness at side
Nose	Prominent	Softness and height at crown

Chin	Square	Long hair
		●
		Hair away from face
		●
	Pointed	Softness and height at crown
		●
		Side part
Neck	Long	Long hair
		●
	Short	Short hair

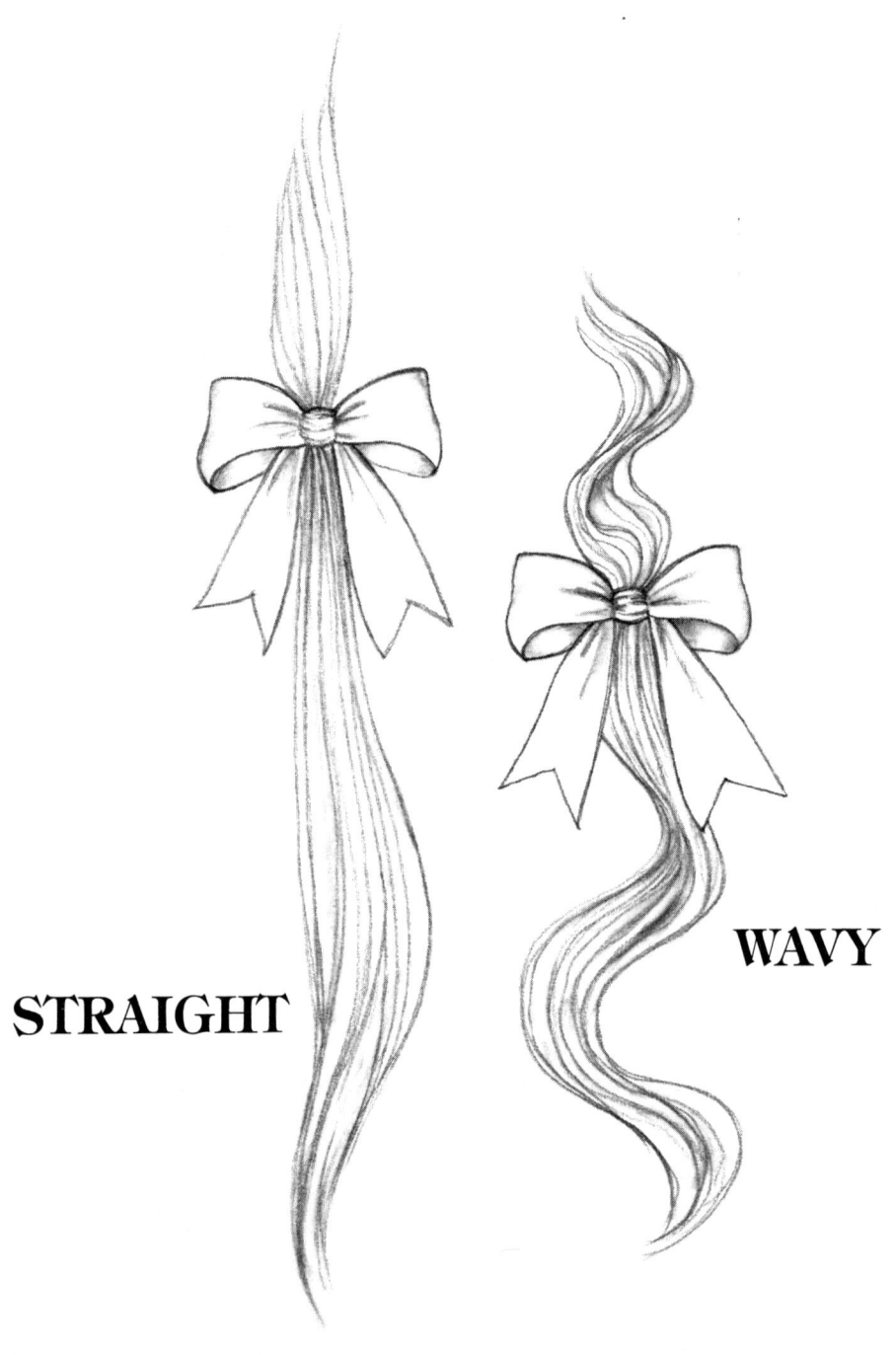

STRAIGHT

WAVY

It will be easier for you and your hairdresser to select the most flattering and manageable hairstyle if you agree on the characteristics of your hair—whether the texture is fine, medium, or coarse, and the quantity thin and sparsely spaced, medium, or thick and full. Determining the amount of curl will also help you select the style that will look terrific from one haircut to the next.

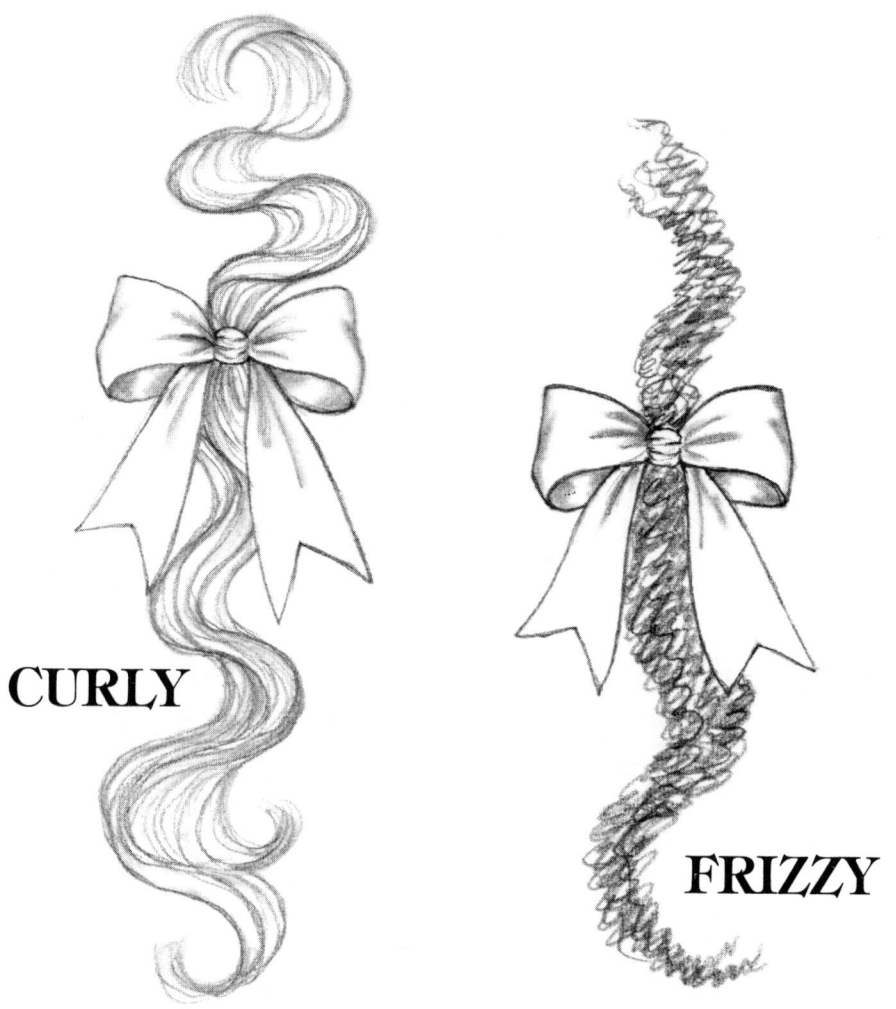

CURLY

FRIZZY

The characteristics described below present certain styling problems. With this information you are now ready to personalize a hairstyle that complements both your features and hair characteristics.

HAIR CHARACTERISTICS	TYPE OF CUT	HOW TO STYLE
Fine	Blunt cut ● Chin length	Body wave ● Heat lamp ● Electric rollers
Thin	Blunt cut ● Short and layered	Body wave ● Blow dryer ● Electric rollers

Frizzy, curly	Short-cropped ● Layered	Air drying ● Massage against the growth pattern
Straight	Shoulder length ● Long (if hair is not fine)	Body perm ● Curling iron ● Crimping iron
Wavy	Chin length ● Layered/blunt cut	Blow dryer ● Crimping iron

Blow-Dry Techniques

- Use a cylindrical, natural bristle or plastic hairbrush for styling.
- Dry and style hair in sections.
- To add fullness, bend from the waist, throw hair forward, and brush from nape of neck to front.
- For curly hair, fluff hair with fingertips while drying; don't brush.
- For oily hair, use a warm, never hot, setting.
- If you blow-dry your hair more than once a week, use a conditioner made especially for use with heat.

Permanents

Permanents will give straight hair soft waves, thin hair more volume, and limp hair more control. The permanents developed for home use are safe and effective if you follow the manufacturer's directions and your hair is neither badly damaged nor chemically treated. With either professional or at-home products, decide beforehand whether you want to add body, waves, or curls to your hair, as the amount of curl you desire determines the type of product needed.

Although they are named permanents, in approximately three to six months the curl will be relaxed. Time and trims are the only way to undo the effects of unwanted or old permanents.

Color

Hair can be colored to add shine, accent highlights, cover gray, or just add excitement to your life. There's a tremendous variety of hair-color products on the market for at-home use, some of which are described below. They are safe if you follow the manufacturer's directions and should result in the desired effect. However, if you're contemplating a severe color change (from brunette to blonde, for example), get a professional job.

FROSTING is bleaching a portion of hair to obtain a salt-and-pepper or streaked look.

HENNA is a natural dye that conditions, shines, and lends body. Except for the natural shade, it adds color and highlights. The natural shade adds highlights only. Fades with repeated washing.

HIGHLIGHTING adds color to random strands of hair to create a shimmering effect.

SHAMPOO-IN-COLOR shampoos, conditions, and colors all in one step.

Problems

The six most common hair problems and what to do about them:

PROBLEM: The frizzies
SYMPTOM: Uncontrollable, unmanageable, and unattractive curling of hair

TREATMENT: Use a conditioner after every shampoo; have hair cut to complement the curls; consider a professional straightening.

PROBLEM: Uncontrollable hair
SYMPTOM: Flyaway hair
TREATMENT: Use cream rinse and conditioner; apply conditioner with fingertips to dry hair; don't use metal brushes or combs.

PROBLEM: Split ends
SYMPTOM: Hair shaft is divided at the end
TREATMENT: The only cure for split ends is to cut them off.

PROBLEM: Dandruff
SYMPTOM: Small, white flakes on the scalp or shoulders
TREATMENT: Use a dandruff shampoo, give scalp a good massage before shampooing, avoid harsh brushing.

PROBLEM: Dull hair
SYMPTOM: No natural shine or luster
TREATMENT: Shampoo and condition hair often; always rinse hair thoroughly. Consider using a highlighting product.

PROBLEM: Thinning hair
SYMPTOM: Greater than normal amount of hair loss
TREATMENT: Avoid brushing; keep hair clean; check with a doctor. A permanent may help hair appear thicker.

Special Effects

Special occasions call for special effects. Add glamour to your hair by curling it tightly, swirling it into a twist or bun, or try the following:

CRIMPED HAIR
- Use a crimping iron and hairpins.
- Take a 1-inch piece of hair, and weave it in and out of the hairpin. Twist ends of pin together. Remove in about an hour.

CORN-ROW BRAIDS
- Gently brush hair up.
- Braid one small section of hair after another making neat parts from one side of the head across the top to the other side. Then braid sections down the back.

Or add fancy combs, flowers, fancy hairpins, scarves, turbans, or fake braids and hairpieces for a dressed-up occasion.

AN IMPORTANT FOCUS

Sparkling healthy eyes are a joy to enhance with the right hairstyle and makeup. The chief rule for keeping them healthy is to have an examination every two years by a doctor, who will test for eye disease as well as fit you for a prescription if need be. If, in addition, you provide your eyes with rest, light, and cleanliness, they will give you much service and little trouble.

REST

- When reading, driving long distances, or watching TV, shut eyes for 30-second spells from time to time.
- Relax with cool, wet cotton pads soaked in water, tea, or witch hazel on eyes.
- Get sufficient sleep. Avoid "all-nighters."
- While doing close work, occasionally look as far away as you can see. Focus eyes on fingers when staring at far-off distances for long periods of time.

LIGHT

- *Always* use plenty of light.
- Wear sunglasses in the sunlight, not indoors. Make sure they are strong enough; if you can see your eyes through the lenses, the glasses aren't of sufficient strength for bright outdoor light. Choose, gray, green, or amber tones for the lenses.
- If you prefer tinted glasses for indoor use, keep the tint weak.

CLEANLINESS

- Remove makeup *every* night.
- Do not lend eye makeup. In fact, this rule applies to all makeup.
- Dispose of used eye makeup over six months old. For this reason it's more economical to purchase eye makeup in small sizes.
- Replace mascara every four months. The moist, dark insides of a mascara tube provide a perfect breeding ground for bacteria and fungi.
- Wash eye brushes, sponges, and applicators frequently.
- Wash glasses in warm water and soap at least twice a week. Soak contact lenses in proper cleansing/soaking solutions.
- If you have oily skin, wipe the bridge of your nose and your glasses with an astringent.

ACCENT ON HANDS

Tools:
- Nail polish remover
- Clippers
- Scissors
- Emery board
- Bath oil
- Nail fortifier

- Nail buffer and cream
- Base coat
- Nail polish
- Sealer or top coat

After the face, hands are the most visible area of skin and can contribute a lot to your attractiveness. Hands respond beautifully to a minimum of care and are worth the attention.

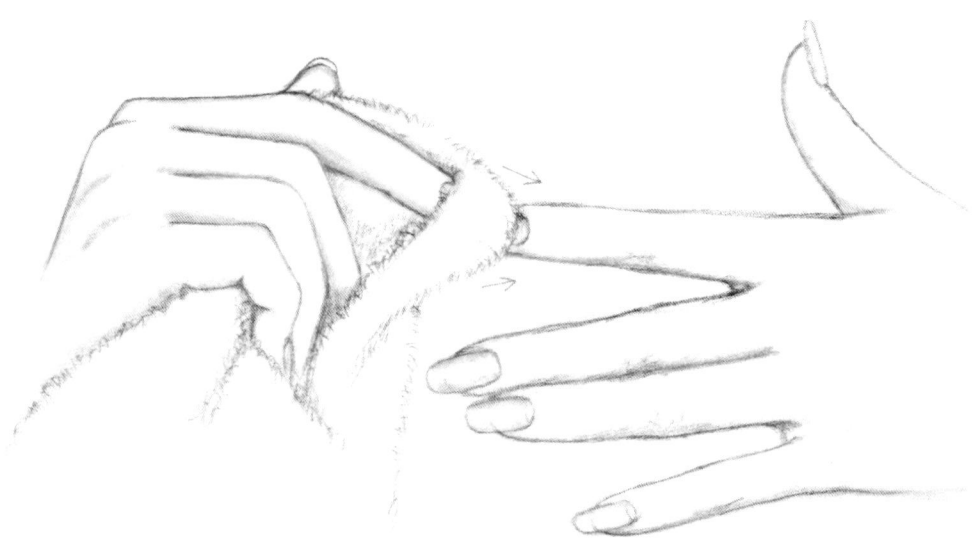

PROTECT

- Lubricate frequently and lavishly with lotion.
- Always lubricate your hands after they touch water.

- Wear lined rubber gloves for wet work.
- Wear cotton gloves for household chores and gardening.
- Push cuticles back with a towel every time you wash your hands to prevent them from becoming rough and broken.
- Wear sun protection on hands.

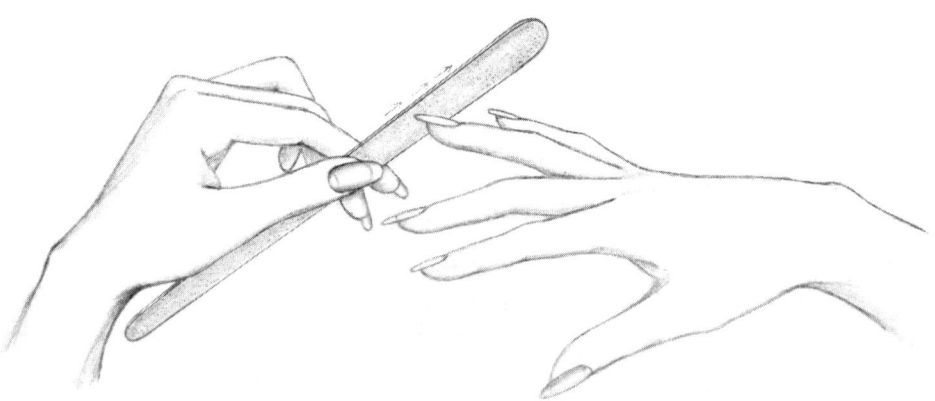

MANICURE

(Once a week)
- Remove all traces of old polish, moving from base to tip of nail.
- Shape nails first with scissors or nail clippers, then an emery board to smooth edges. File in one direction only.
- Soak nails for five minutes in warm water with oil added (either bath or baby oil).
- Push back cuticles with a towel after drying. Massage cuticles with cream.

- Trim hangnails with scissors.
- Moving from base to tip, apply nail fortifier, base coat, one to two coats of polish, and a top coat. Make sure nail is thoroughly dry between applications.

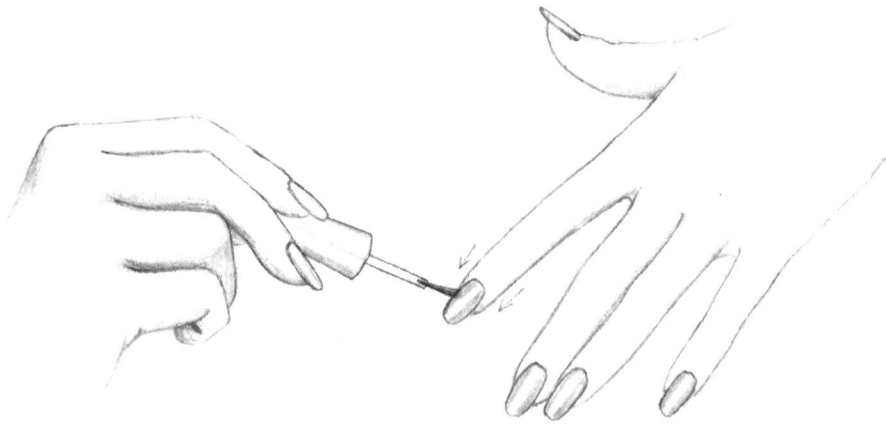

MAINTENANCE

- Reapply a nail sealer or top coat every two or three days.
- Touch up chipped polish on tips of nails.
- Buff nails between polishings; use a nail buffer or chamois cloth. Apply some nail cream and buff in one direction until nail gleams. Stop if nail feels warm.
- If nail chips or breaks, purchase a nail-mending kit or cut all nails down to the same size.

Tips

- Use cotton swabs to remove polish from sides of nails.
- Use nail polish remover no more than twice a week, as it dries out the nail surface.

- Use a pencil to dial a phone.
- Set polish after it has dried by immersing fingertips in cold water for a few seconds.
- Remember that nails are stronger and less liable to break if kept to a smooth oval shape rather than a pointed dagger.
- If nails tend to break, use a polish with added hardeners.
- Use clear polish for a quick shine.

IF YOU BITE YOUR NAILS . . .
- Get a professional manicure and see if you want to destroy all that work.
- Learn to knit or embroider.
- Buy a "worry" stone that you can play with while talking.
- In extreme cases, consult a professional hypnotist.

SEE a DOCTOR IF . . .
- Bumps or ridges occur on nail.
- Any discoloration appears.
- Excessive breakage occurs.

ACCENT ON FEET

Tools:
- Nail polish remover
- Nail clippers
- Bath oil or foot soak
- Pumice stone
- Nail fortifier
- Cuticle cream
- Base coat
- Nail polish
- Sealer or top coat

Perhaps because feet are so far from our eyes we tend to neglect them. Many women give their hands consistent attention and weekly manicures, yet splash a layer of color on their toenails whenever they notice the previous color has chipped off and call it a pedicure. Proper foot care is essential to prevent problems and guarantees us a long life of brisk walking.

There are probably very few women who haven't gone through a night of stylish misery wearing a pair of uncomfortable but oh so fashionable shoes. You may think the strain doesn't show, but the tense way you move and the tightness in your face give you away and detract from the rest of your attractive look. First and above all in foot care, *please* buy shoes that fit properly and feel comfortable!

If you consistently abuse your feet, you will sooner or later find yourself in orthopedic shoes with a real set of physical problems—a high price to pay for looking stylish.

Foot care, like hand care, works in three stages: protection, pedicure, and maintenance.

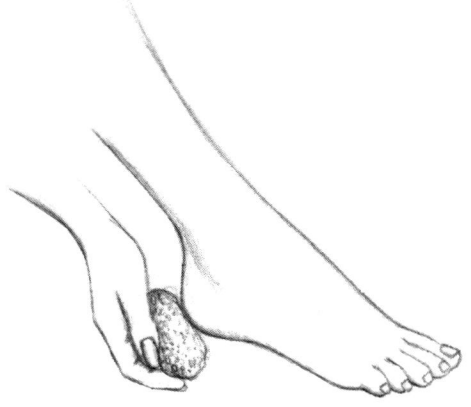

PROTECT

- Cleanse thoroughly in the tub or shower with a loofah and plenty of soap.
- Use a pumice stone on heels and calluses.
- Wear clean peds, socks, stockings, or panty hose with closed shoes and sneakers.
- Powder the inside of your shoes before wearing them.
- Give extra lubrication to rough spots before retiring at night.

PEDICURE

1. Remove all traces of old polish, moving from base to tip of nail.

2. Shape nails into a square by clipping them straight across with toenail clippers.
3. Soak feet for five minutes in warm water and oil, or a specially prepared foot soak.
4. Rub calluses and heels with a pumice stone and rinse off dead skin.
5. Push back cuticles with a towel after drying. Massage with cuticle cream.

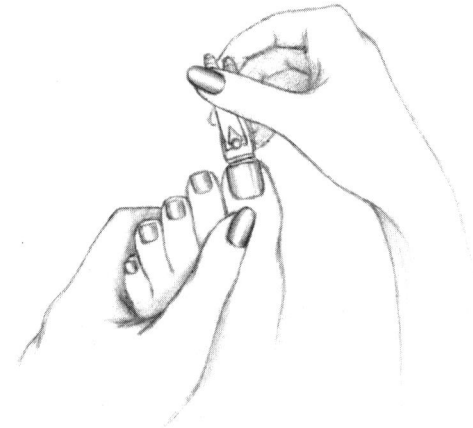

6. Trim hangnails with clippers.
7. Moving from base to tip, apply nail fortifier, base coat, one to two coats of polish, and a top coat. Make sure nails are thoroughly dry between applications.

MAINTENANCE

- Exercise feet: Walk on tiptoe, flex feet and point toes, go barefoot in the house.
- Switch shoes from day to day, during the day if possible.
- Have someone massage your feet.
- Change socks often.
- Keep feet warm in the winter.

Tips

- Soak tired feet in a warm baking soda solution.
- Revitalize circulation by alternately immersing feet in hot, then cold soaks for 10 minutes.
- Try a charcoal shoe liner to absorb foot odor.
- Wear cotton or wool socks rather than nylon.

SEE a DOCTOR IF . . .

. . . You have corns or calluses.

. . . Bumps or ridges occur on the nail.

. . . Toenails begin growing into the skin.

. . . Hard painful lumps begin to appear in the skin.

. . . Any discoloration of the nail or foot appears.

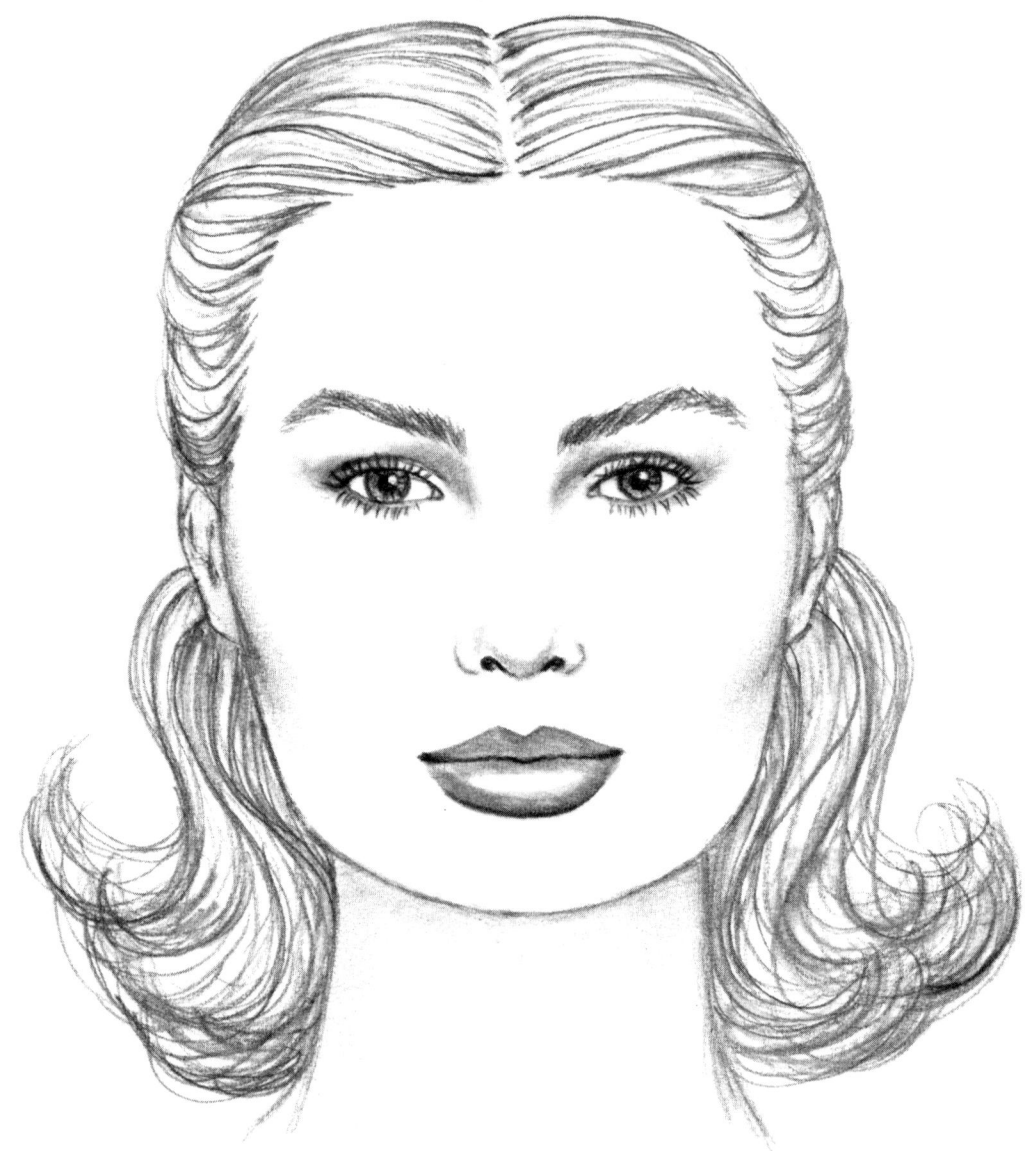

Makeover #1

FLAWS

1. Unflattering hairstyle for square face
2. Thick eyebrows
3. Small eyes
4. Wide cheeks
5. Square jaw
6. Bottom lip too full
7. Receding chin

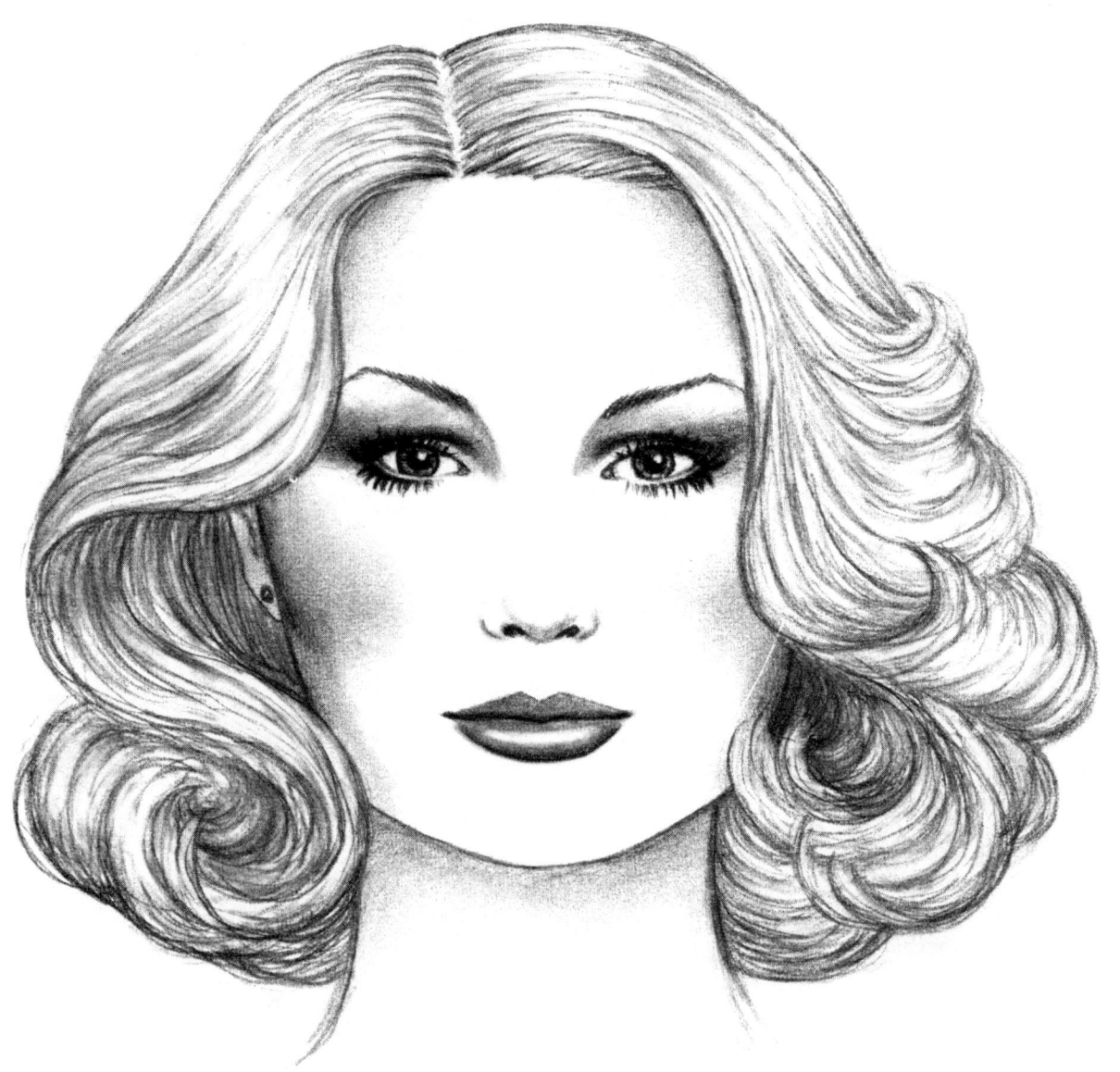

CORRECTIONS

1. Soften angles of hairstyle.
2. Reshape brows.
3. Enlarge eyes.
4. Narrow cheeks through contouring.
5. Soften angle of jaw through contouring.
6. Reshape lip.
7. Highlight chin area.

Illustrated Makeover #1

1. The hairstyle is very unflattering for a square face. The facial angles have been softened with a side-swept part and a fluff at the jawline. Limp or thin hair may require a body permanent to accomplish this.

2. The eyebrows were too bushy and distracting. They were tweezed across the bridge of the nose and then brushed up with an eyebrow brush-comb. All straggly hairs have been removed.

3. Small eyes can made to look larger by adding a pale shadow to the eyelid and a darker shadow in the crease. A dot of white shadow or highlighter should be applied directly under the brow.

4. The wide cheeks now appear narrower through the use of darker foundation. When contouring is applied down the sides of the cheeks, it appears to contract the width of the cheeks.

5. The square jawline of this model has been corrected with the use of a concealer or a darker foundation applied to the sides. Be sure to blend the edges.

6. The lower lip can be made to appear less full by camouflaging it with foundation and powder, then redrawing the lower lipline with a lip brush just to the inside of the natural lipline.

7. The receding chin on this model appears less conspicuous when highlighter is applied to the entire area. The addition of cheek color over this area tends to intensify the chin.

Illustrated Makeover #2

1. The hairstyle is too long for the amount of curl in the hair. Keeping the hair at a shorter length will give it more uniformity and shape and distract less from the face

2. The eyebrows are overly tweezed and look unnatural. They should be allowed to grow back to their natural shape, tweezing only the few strav hairs under the arch. In the meantime, they have been filled in with eyebrow pencil.

3. The short nose now appears longer through the use of highlighter applied down the sides of the nose.

4. The droopy lids are made less prominent by using a light shadow along the inner half of the upper lid and a dark shadow along the outer half. Dark, matted shadow is applied where lids begin to droop, highlighter dotted under inner edge of brow, eyeliner used from inner top edge to pupil of eye.

5. The crooked mouth of the model has been corrected by applying foundation over lips and dusting with powder. With the lip brush, the upper and lower lips are redrawn to appear straight. The outline has been filled in with lipstick applied directly from the tube.

6. The pointed chin has been corrected by contouring the area with darker foundation to soften the angle.

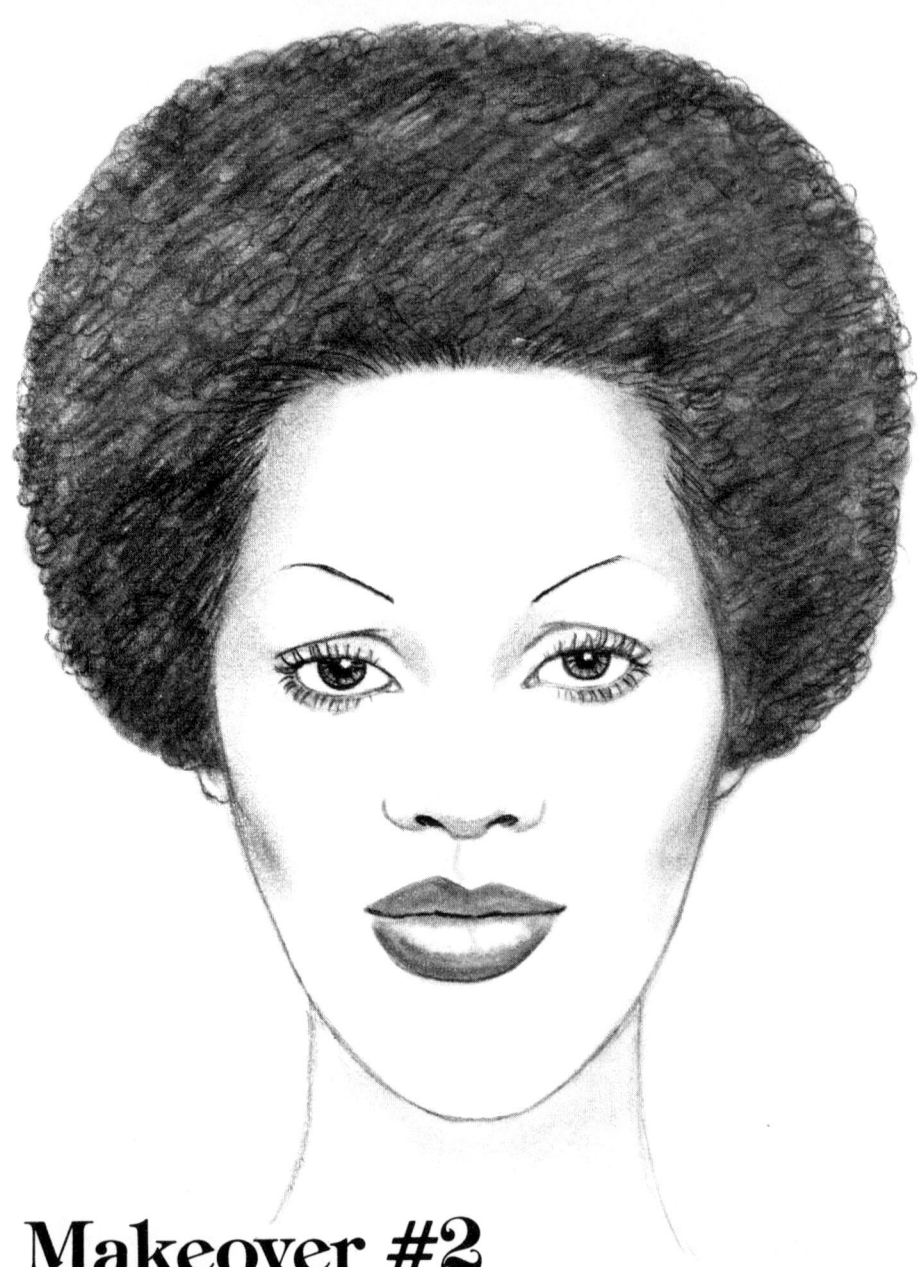

Makeover #2
FLAWS

1. Hair too long for hair type
2. Overly tweezed eyebrows
3. Short nose
4. Droopy lids
5. Crooked mouth
6. Pointed chin

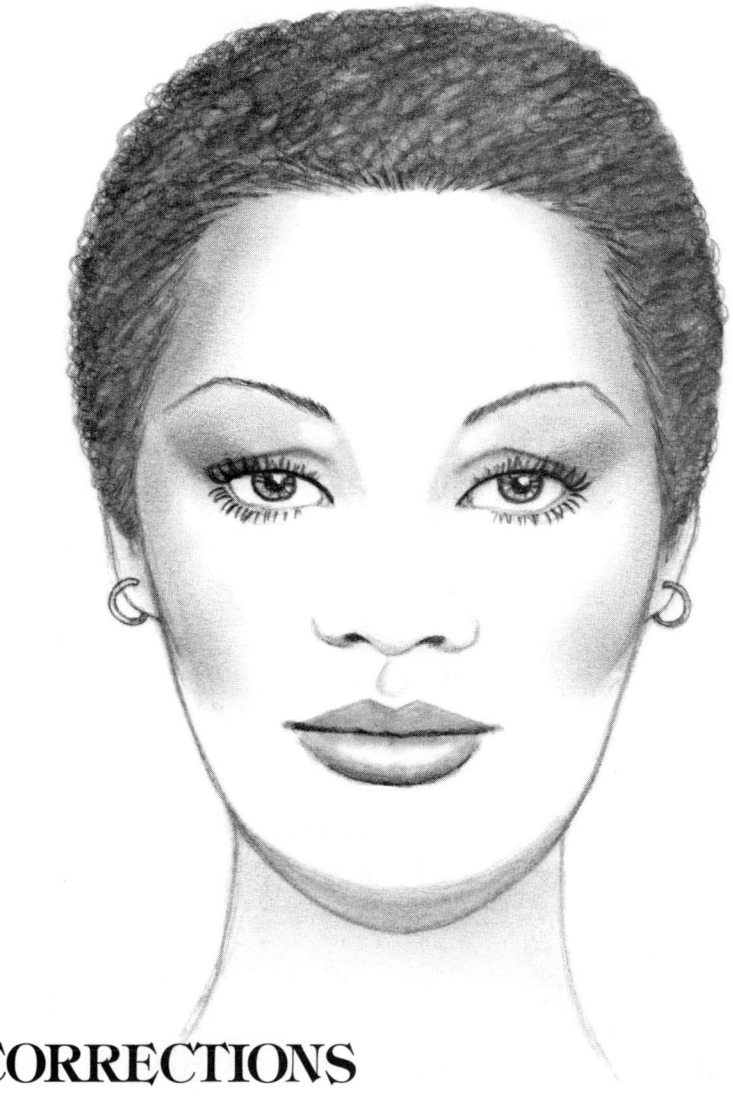

CORRECTIONS

1. Keep hair shorter
2. Shape eyebrows with pencil.
3. Lengthen nose with highlighter.
4. Minimize lids with shadow.
5. Reshape lips.
6. Contouring applied to chin.

THE FRAME GAME

There was a time when women avoided wearing glasses at the price of not seeing. Today, some people can even be found purchasing glasses filled with clear, nonprescriptive lenses in an effort to appear stylish, for glasses have become a fashion accessory as well as an aid to good vision. As with all other forms of style, the fashion in glasses changes too. For example, the metal frames that were so popular in the early 1970s have been replaced by large, light plastic frames. But what has not changed are basic principles that can accent good features or alter facial imbalances.

Women who wear glasses should never forget makeup, especially on the eyes. It is not a general rule that you need to wear more eye makeup; only those with thick lenses or those with a prescription for myopia need to wear a little more. The color of your frames, like your makeup, should be selected according to hair and skin tones. A number of cosmetic firms are providing a complete, coordinated line of makeup to match eyeglass frames.

The process of frame selection is not as complicated as you might think when you first are confronted with such an array of frames. Just use this chart to match your facial shape and features to the most flattering frame shapes, bridges, and colors.

FACIAL CHARACTERISTICS		FRAME TYPE
Facial shape	Long or narrow	Square •
		Round •
		Wide •
		Wide on top •
		Straight lower rim •
	Oval	Any shape •

FACIAL CHARACTERISTICS		FRAME TYPE
Facial shape	Square	Wide square ● Rectangular ● Round
	Round	Oval ● Square ● Elliptical
	Triangle	Wide top ● Narrow bottom ● Shallow rectangles ● Aviator

Nose Narrow
 •
 Long
 •
 Broad Saddle bridge
 • •
 Turned up Pads that rest on
  nose to support
 • glasses
  •
 Short High-bridged

SKIN TONES	COLOR OF FRAME
Fair/pale	Pastels, beige, pale plum, blue, green, pale brown
Sallow	Blue, blue-green, violet, wine, brown, red
Pink/ruddy	Gold, amber, honey, gray, blue
Olive	Peach, brown, red and pink, plum, gold
Dark/black	Plum, wine, gold, intense and bright colors, brown, black, navy

Tips

- Spend time studying yourself before you buy.
- Look at yourself in your new frames in a full-length mirror as well as a short mirror before purchasing.
- Consult the optometrist for a correct fit.

CONTACT LENSES

The advantages of both hard and soft lenses are the following:

•

Truer vision with no distortion.

•

Improved peripheral vision.

•

No clouding from temperature changes.

•

No breakage of frames.

•

Some stabilization of prescription.

•

Hard lenses take a few weeks and some determination to adjust to, but are well worth the effort. Soft lenses require less adjustment time than hard lenses but require more maintenance. Your doctor will advise you about the type of lens that is suitable for you.

Regardless of the kind you use, contact lens wearers should know the following restrictions concerning makeup:

- Insert soft lenses before applying any eye makeup.
- Insert hard lenses when it suits you during application of makeup.
- Cream shadows are recommended for lens wearers. If you prefer powdered shadows, apply them very, very carefully and sparingly.
- Frosted shadows are not recommended; the specks have a tendency to get lodged under the lenses.
- Use makeup remover after removing lenses, never before.
- Do not apply liner on inner margin of lid. This is a great technique, but one lens wearers must sacrifice.

- Do not use cotton balls to remove makeup, as fibers cling to lashes. Pressed cotton pads or tissues are preferable.
- Do not use lash-lengthening mascaras with fibers.
- Do not use hair sprays and perfume sprays while wearing lenses. If you must, shut your eyes tightly and leave the room quickly when through.
- Be wary of eyedrops. Consult your doctor before their use.

FASHIONING YOUR WARDROBE

Understanding a few of the basic principles of line in dress can help you to create a more flattering wardrobe to go with your prettier face and perfect hairstyle. Once you have decided which areas you want to accentuate and which you would rather camouflage, check with the chart to see how the structure of a dress can help you.

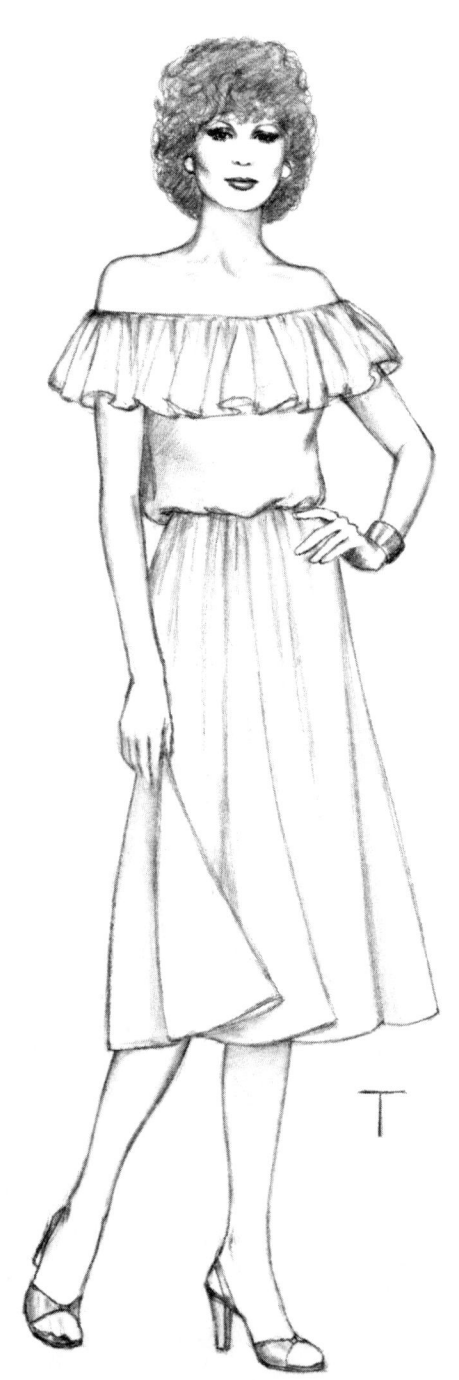

- A T-line creates an illusion of being shorter.
- The eye is drawn from the bottom up and then across.
- Great for the slim and tall figure.

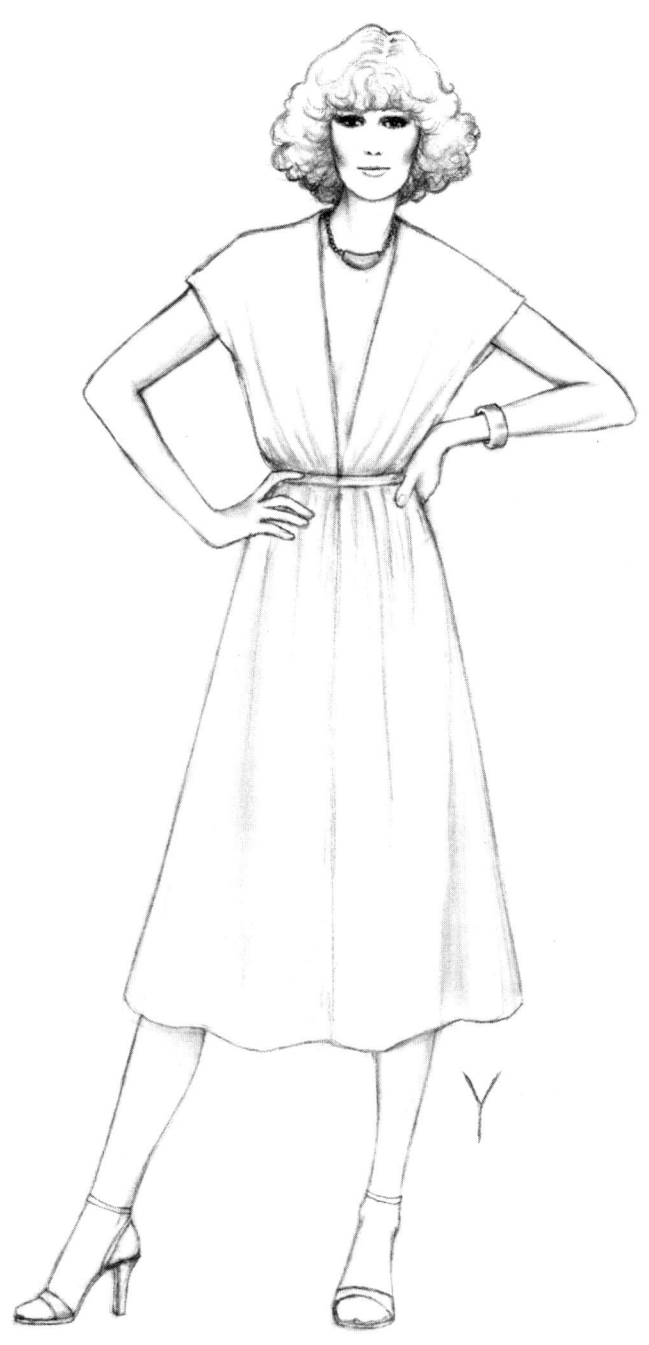

- A Y-line creates an illusion of height.
- The eye is drawn from the bottom up and keeps on going.
- Great for the shorter figure.

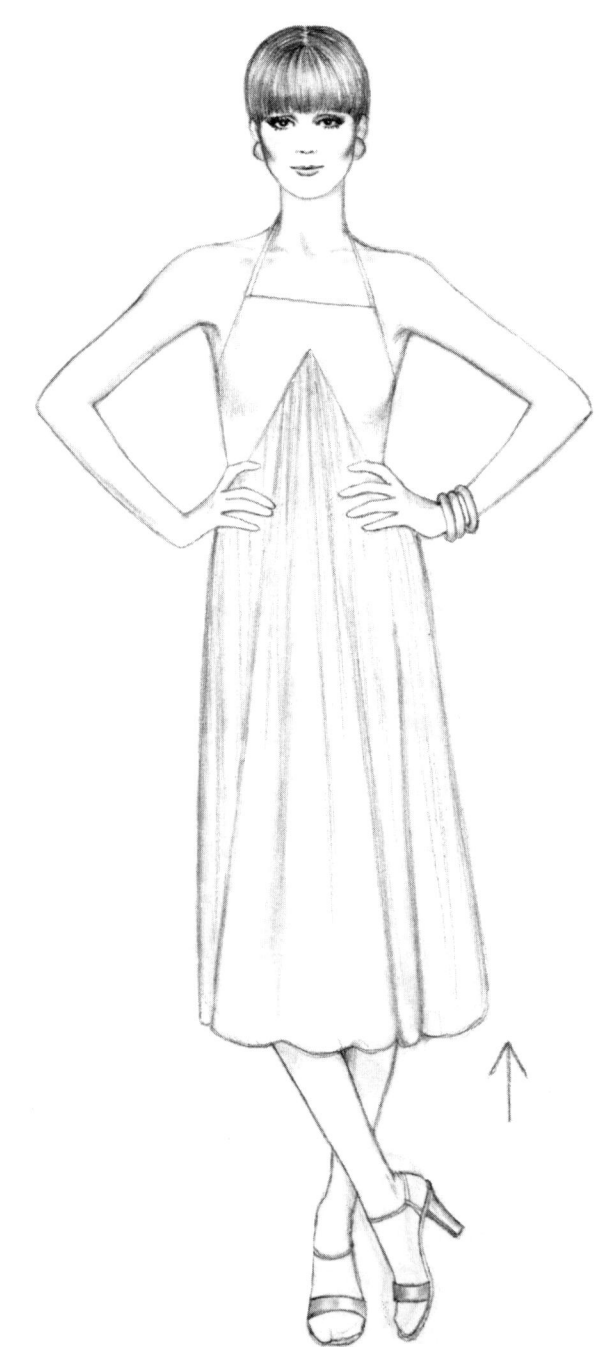

- A pyramid-line creates an illusion of being short.
- The eye is drawn from the bottom up and then back down again.
- Great for the tall figure.

- A I-line creates an illusion of height.
- The eye is drawn from the bottom up and keeps on going.
- Great for the shorter figure.

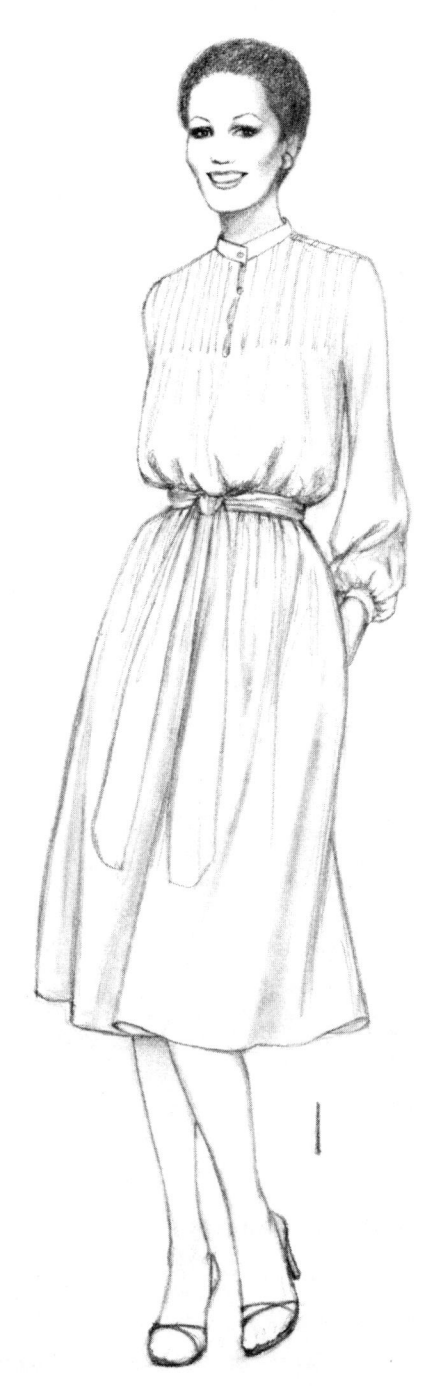

The design, texture, and color of a fabric are other important factors in selecting clothing that will accentuate or camouflage.

IF YOU WANT TO APPEAR:	THEN CHOOSE THESE:	AND AVOID THESE:
TALLER	Vertical stripes • Diagonal stripes	Horizontal stripes
SLIMMER	Dark colors • Small prints	Bright colors Large, bold prints
SHORTER	Horizontal stripes	Vertical stripes

IF YOU WANT TO APPEAR:	THEN CHOOSE THESE:	AND AVOID THESE:
HEAVIER	Nubby fabrics • Large prints • Large plaids • Bright colors • Horizontal stripes • Shiny fabrics	Vertical stripes • Small prints • Smooth fabrics • Dark colors

Let the five Fs of fashion be your guide in selecting your wardrobe:

● FUNCTIONAL

Function is the foremost reason for buying a garment. Whether you are dressing for warmth or a special event, make sure the garment is appropriate, because if it does not suit its primary purpose, it may just sit in your closet.

● FLEXIBLE

Your clothing will be worth more if you purchase flexible items. Is the garment versatile? Can it be worn in the office by day, and with a change of accessories be ready for dinner that evening? Can it be worn from one season into the next? Your clothes should be as flexible as you are.

● FASHIONABLE

To be fashionable does not mean that you must conform to a certain mode, for fashion today is the extension of a woman's personality and life-style. Clothes should make a statement about who you are, how you feel about yourself, and how you live your life.

● FIT

Loose or clingy, the garment you choose must fit correctly. Ill-fitting clothes are uncomfortable and detract from your appearance, so observe how the following areas fit when selecting a garment:
● Neck
● Shoulder
● Bust
● Waistline
● Sleeve length
● Sleeve width
● Crotch
● Hemline

- FUN

If an outfit follows the first four Fs and also gives you pleasure and enjoyment, then you know it's right. Whether for jogging or an evening out, your clothes should say that you're glad to be you.

Tips

- Selection of the correct undergarments is the foundation for clothes that fit properly.
- Always repair a torn hem, a missing button, or a ripped seam.
- Clean, well-cared-for clothes are no accident. Launder and dry-clean as necessary.
- No longer do the strict rules of color apply; be expressive!

BODY TONICS

The right clothes for your height and body build will look even more attractive when you have the healthiest, firmest body to wear them on. That body is based on the food you put into it. We don't believe in desperate diets. We believe in eating sensibly. Unless you have an upset metabolism, allergies, or a specific physical problem, proper food intake will eventually bring you to your best weight, supply you with energy, keep your body in smooth working order, and aid in good health maintenance. Selection of the right foods can sometimes be a confusing process, as experts' impressive new claims about certain foods seem to crop up monthly, only to be destroyed later by other experts' research. It's wiser to stick to fundamentals, like the Basic Four as a guideline.

The Basic Four

PROTEIN GROUP
(two servings daily)
Meat, poultry, fish, shellfish, eggs, dried beans or peas, soybeans, lentils, nuts, cheese, brewer's yeast

GRAINS GROUP
(four servings daily)
Grains, especially whole wheat and rye breads, cereals, rice, cornmeal

FRUIT/VEGETABLE GROUP
(four servings daily)
All fruits and vegetables, especially green and yellow vegetables, citrus fruits

DAIRY PRODUCTS
(one or two servings daily)
Milk, yogurt, cheese, cottage cheese

The size of the serving depends upon your size and appetite. The variety of foods that you select from the Basic Four will provide you with the daily necessary nutrients.

Necessary Nutrients

	USE	FOUND IN
Proteins	Build and repair tissue ● Tone muscle ● Maintain skin	Meat, poultry fish, shellfish, eggs, soybeans, dried pies, lentils, nuts, cheese, brewer's yeast, beans

	USE	FOUND IN
Carbohydrates	Provide energy ● Aid in digestion	Grains, cereals, breads, molasses, potatoes, rice, fresh fruits and vegetables, alcoholic beverages
Fats	Provide energy ● Lubricate skin ● Aid in vitamin absorption	Animal foods, butter, oils, nuts, cheeses, whole milk
Minerals	Trigger and maintain system's functioning	Most foods, especially milk, shellfish, green vegetables Essential to survival

	USE	FOUND IN
Water	Essential to survival ● (drink six glasses daily)	

    Some foods are superior to others. Healthy food furnishes lots of nutrients and roughage in an unadulterated form. The unhealthy foods are loaded with excessive fats, artificial additives, refined carbohydrates, salt, or sugar. Excessive fats cause a buildup of excess cholesterol, which can lead to heart disease. The case for the connection between artificial additives and some forms of cancer becomes stronger every day. Refined carbohydrates, like white flour, have been stripped of much of their nutrients by modern food-processing techniques. Too much salt has been associated with the onset of hypertension and unnecessary water retention. Refined sugar creates dental cavities, utilizes a large amount of B vitamins in its digestion, and uses the body's supply of insulin too quickly, making you crave more sugar. Some foods should be avoided, and the list below will help you.

Healthy Foods	Unhealthy Foods
Fresh vegetables, fresh fruits	Sausage, hot dogs, bacon
juices	Pretzels, potato chips, buttered or salted popcorn
Eggs	Olives, pickles
Cheese	Fast foods that have been processed in any way
Yogurt	Fried foods
Skim milk	Chocolate, candy, jelly
Broiled fish	Ice cream
Brewer's yeast	Carbonated sodas
Sprouts	TV dinners
Wheat germ	Beverages containing caffeine
Herbal teas	Alcohol

10 Tips for Overweights
- Put portions on smaller plates.
- Discard top slice of bread, and eat sandwiches open-faced.
- Have a hot drink or soup before meals.
- Eat lots of salad as your first course, but not lots of creamy salad dressing.

- Eat slowly, take small bites, chew food thoroughly, put fork down between mouthfuls.
- If you can't control yourself at restaurants, don't go.
- Take seconds on healthy food (like vegetables).
- Take emergency snack food with you (like fruit).
- Don't wander into the kitchen.
- Join a club for overweights.

10 Tips for Underweights
- Relax before eating.
- Don't let snacks interfere with your meals.
- Eat at least three meals a day.
- Eat your main course first.
- Prepare food in an appetizing way.
- Set a nice table; enjoy your meal.
- Eat breakfast!
- Make thick milkshakes with egg, milk, and bananas.
- Add powdered milk, wheat germ or brewer's yeast to as many foods or drinks as you can.
- Remember: Thin is healthy.

10 Tips for Everyone
- Eat every meal, especially breakfast.
- Do not keep junk foods in the house.
- Be conscious of what you eat.
- Eat at a slow, relaxed pace.

- Decorate your table and make meals pleasant.
- Snack on fresh fruits and fresh vegetables.
- Use foods packed in water, not syrup or oils.
- Chew sugarless gum, if you must chew at all.
- Alternate club soda with alcoholic drinks.
- Ignore weight charts. You know when you feel good.

BODY TONERS

Forget the weight charts, don't bother with pinching your body to see how much fat you can or cannot grab, don't bunch your skin into a big bulge and count the dimples. Just take off your clothes and stand in front of a mirror (preferably a three-way mirror) under a strong light and look at yourself, the whole you from top to bottom, front to back, section by section, and then an overall view. Does it please you? Don't worry about being too fat or thin. Think instead in terms of the following:

- Proportion. Do undesirable parts of your body protrude?
- Muscle tone. Do you have soft, flabby areas or firm, solid ones?
- Skin Tone. Does your skin have a nice, smooth, healthy glow or a bumpy, pimply, dull-looking surface?

It's easy to correct any problems that you see. Honestly. A program of sensible eating along with exercise *has* to produce a healthy, attractive body. In addition to improving appearance and firming muscles, did you know that exercise can

- Improve circulation and heart action
- Induce more restful sleep
- Increase energy
- Help prevent disease
- Increase general stamina
- Make you feel great
- Relax you more than a martini
- Decrease feelings of stress
- Boost your self-confidence
- Increase body awareness

Don't Move

Analyze your posture. Are you sitting up straight? Holding yourself correctly is the quickest body improvement there is. Proper posture means that your

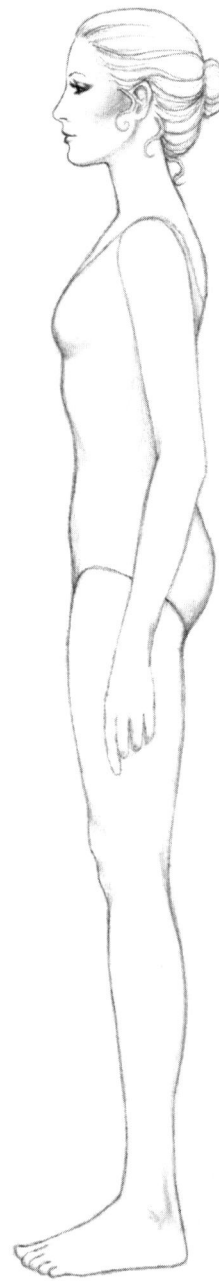

- head is centered over spine
- neck is straight
- shoulders are back and relaxed
- chest is up
- stomach is pulled in and up
- buttocks are tucked in
- knees are slightly bent
- weight of body is resting on both feet

Concentrate on good posture until it becomes a habit.

Spot Exercises

Develop the habit of exercise. Three days of spot exercising with two days of sport exercising every week will improve and maintain your figure; of course you can work out more. Devise your own program by selecting at least one spot exercise from each group, then adding a few extra ones for your trouble areas.

Tips

- Wear a leotard. Better yet, wear nothing.
- Always use the floor, never the bed or sofa.
- Don't exercise on a full stomach.
- Breathe and move in a steady rhythm.
- Relax your face as you move.
- Use music or the TV to accompany you if you wish.

TO WARM UP AND COOL DOWN

Start and end with the "Hymn to the Sun." It's a graceful movement adapted from yoga that stretches all your muscles. Complete each movement as you are inhaling or exhaling.

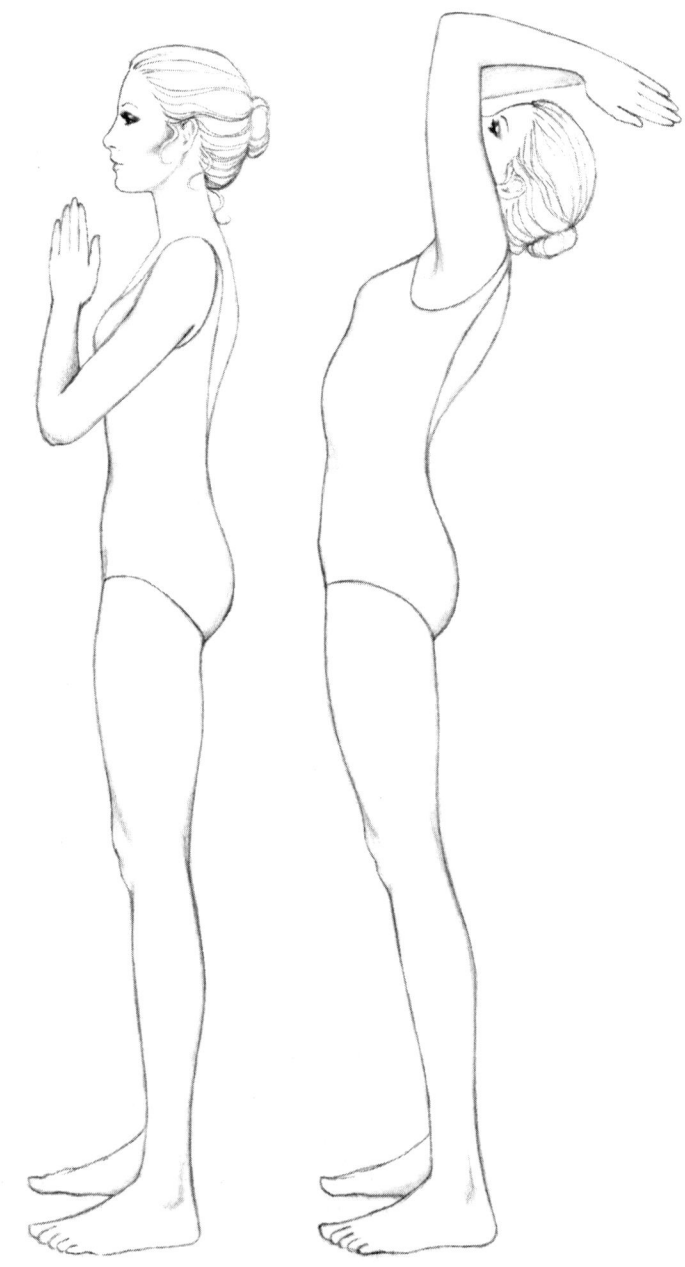

1. Stand up straight, legs, together, hands in prayer position in front of chest.
2. Inhale deeply— raise arms up and over head, extending them back as far as possible.

3. Exhale—separate hands and reach forward as far as possible. Keep reaching till hands touch floor.

4. Inhale—squat with head erect and left leg extended straight out backward.

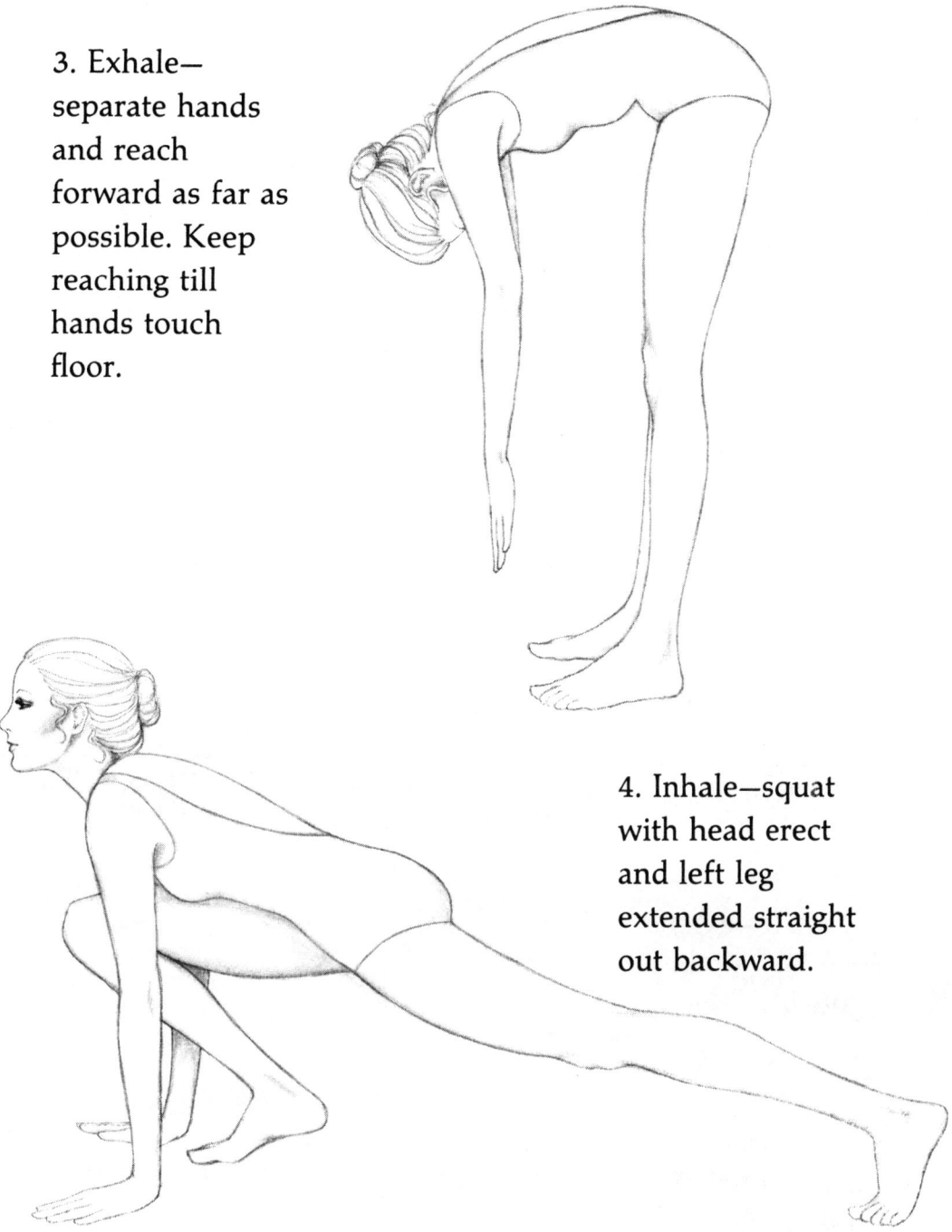

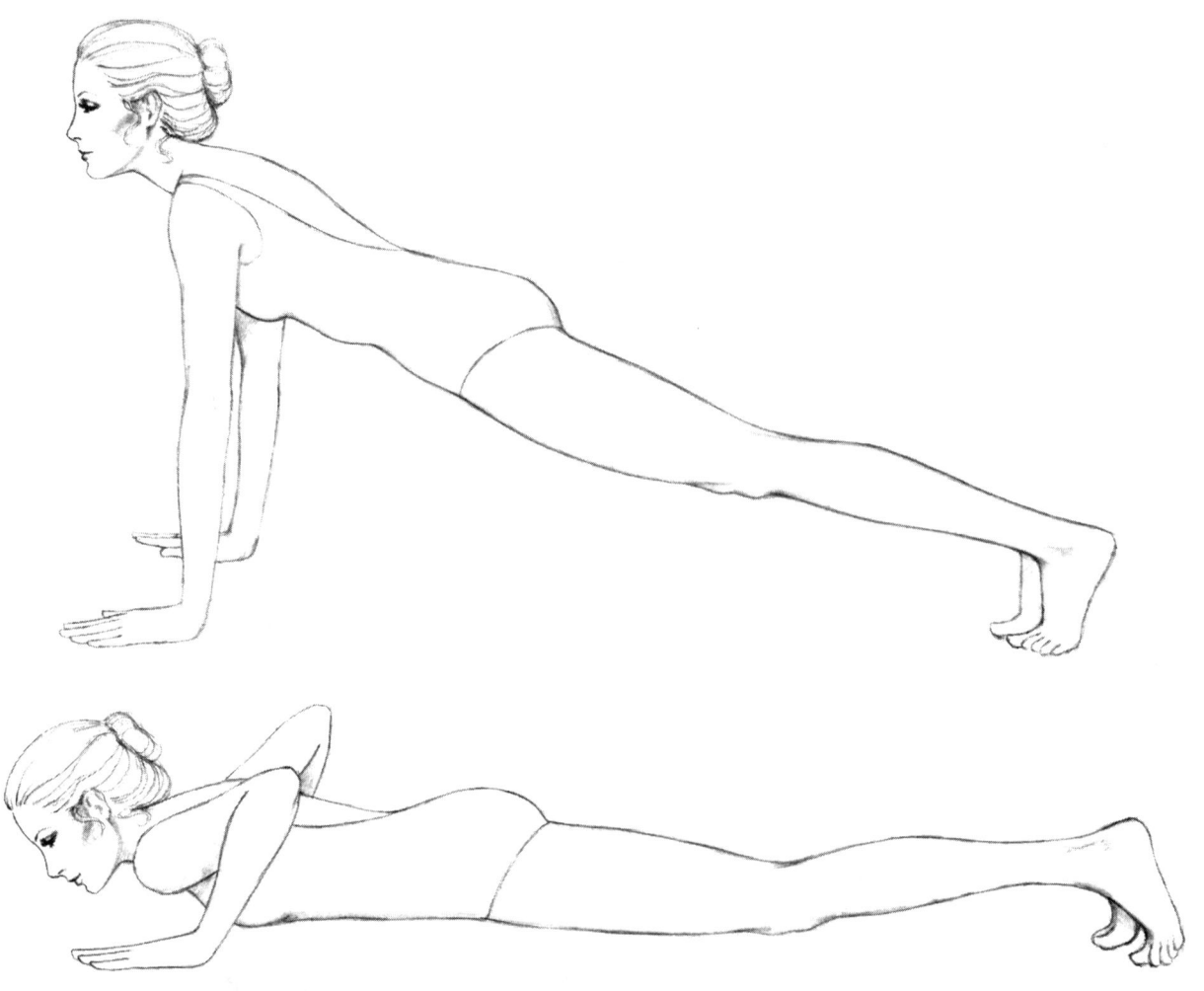

5. Exhale—extend right leg out so body is supported by hands and toes. Lower body down till you are lying on floor.

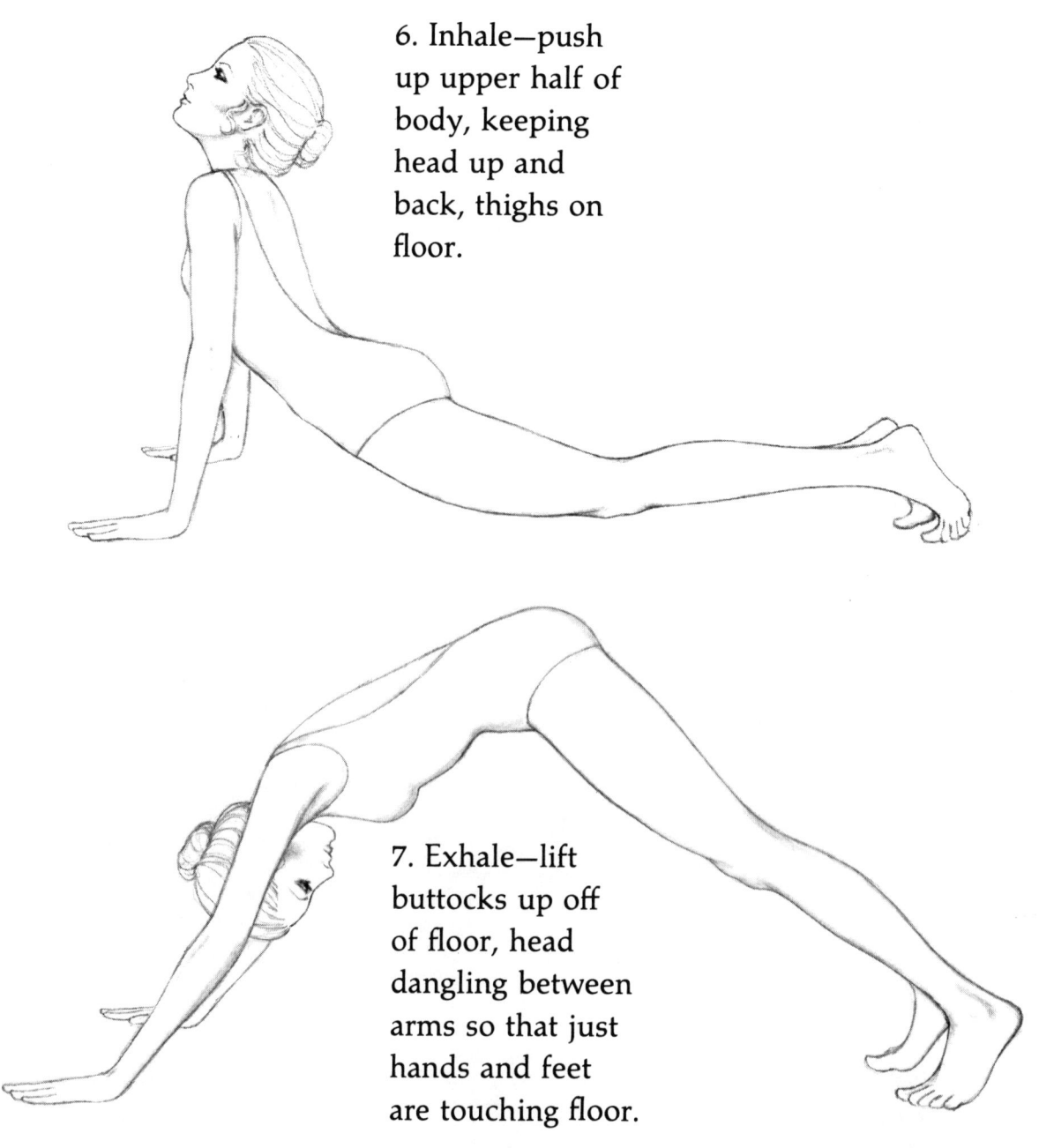

6. Inhale—push up upper half of body, keeping head up and back, thighs on floor.

7. Exhale—lift buttocks up off of floor, head dangling between arms so that just hands and feet are touching floor.

8. Inhale—return to squatting position, now with left leg bent and right leg extended.

9. Exhale—keep hands on floor, bring feet together and straighten legs.

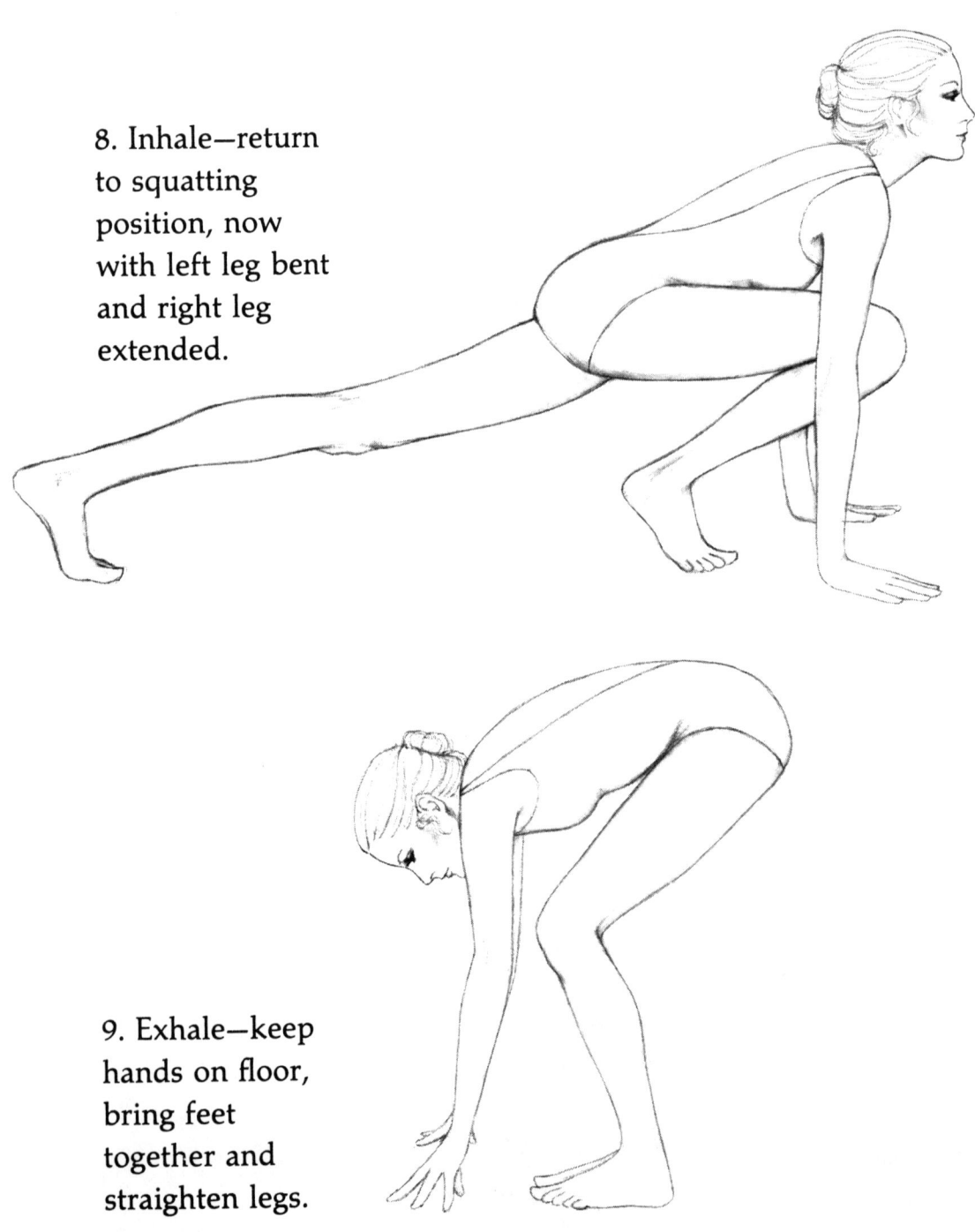

10. Inhale—straighten up with arms extended back over head.

11. Exhale—and return to prayer position.

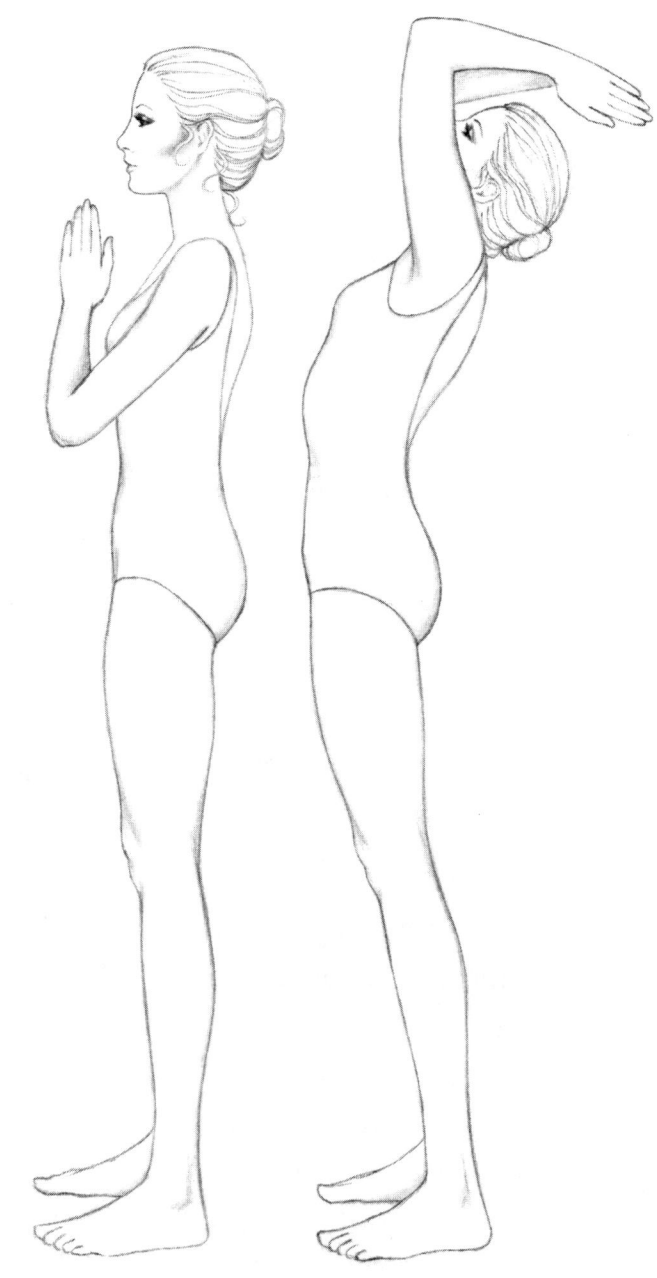

Two other warm-up exercises:
1. Stand straight, tighten buttocks together, hold in tummy hard for 10 seconds.
2. Bend halfway over and dangle head loosely in front of body.

NECK AND CHIN

1. Roll neck slowly around in a complete circle. Change to other direction. Repeat twice.
2. Sit or stand straight. Throw head back, open mouth wide. Close mouth by pulling chin up to mouth. Repeat 10 times.

BUST AND ARMS

1. Stand straight, grasp forearms with hands and push hard for 10 seconds.
2. Stand with legs slightly apart. Extend arms out straight at sides, and slowly rotate them in increasingly larger circles up to 10 counts. Make circles smaller as you reverse direction.
3. Stand with legs slightly apart. Clasp hands in front of chest, elbows pointed out. Push air away from chest, extending arms straight in front of you. Return to original position. Repeat 10 times.

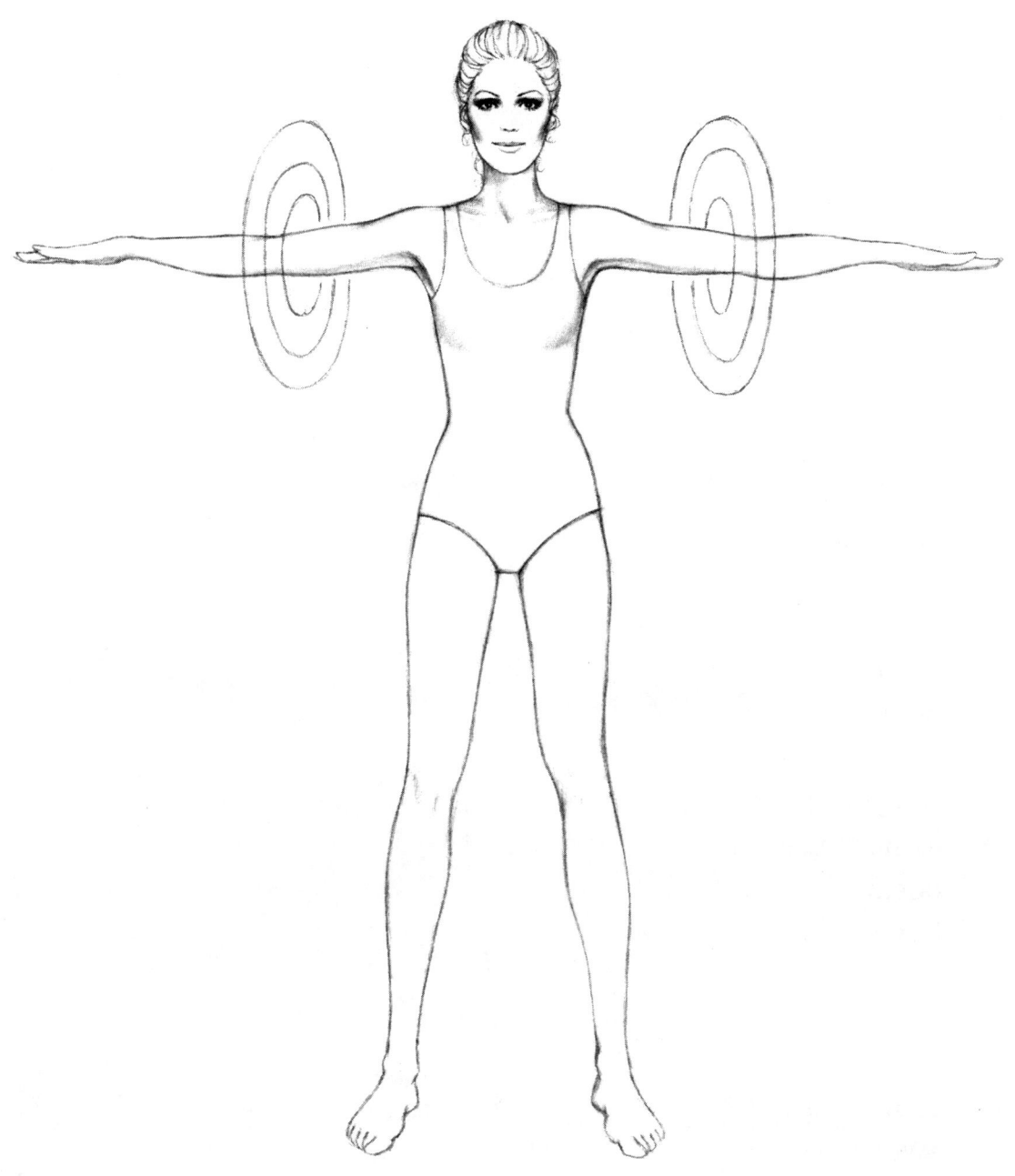

WAIST AND TORSO

1. Stand with legs slightly apart, hands on hips. Lean forward until back is parallel to floor. Swing torso to right side. Swing backwards as far as you can without straining. Swing to left side and back to starting position. Repeat three times, and reverse direction for four complete swings.

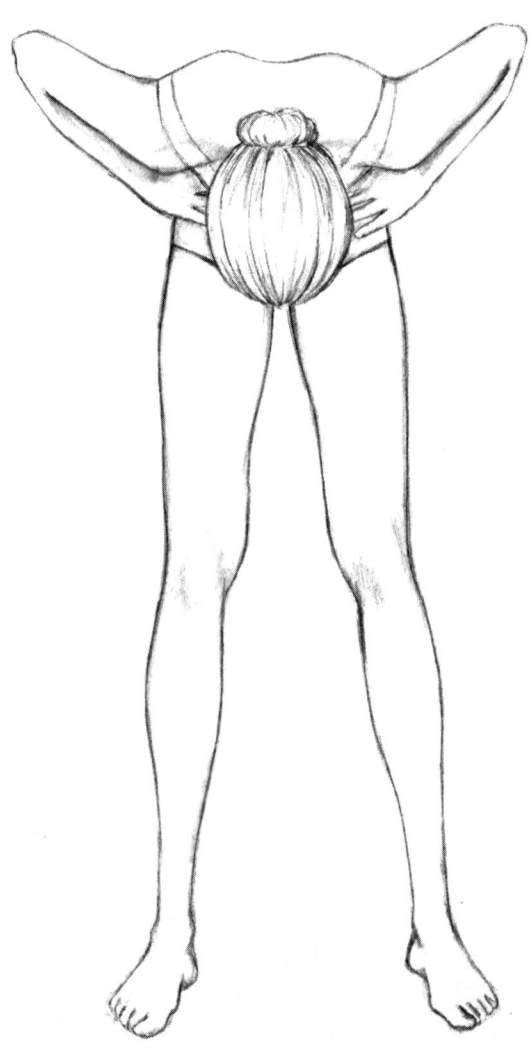

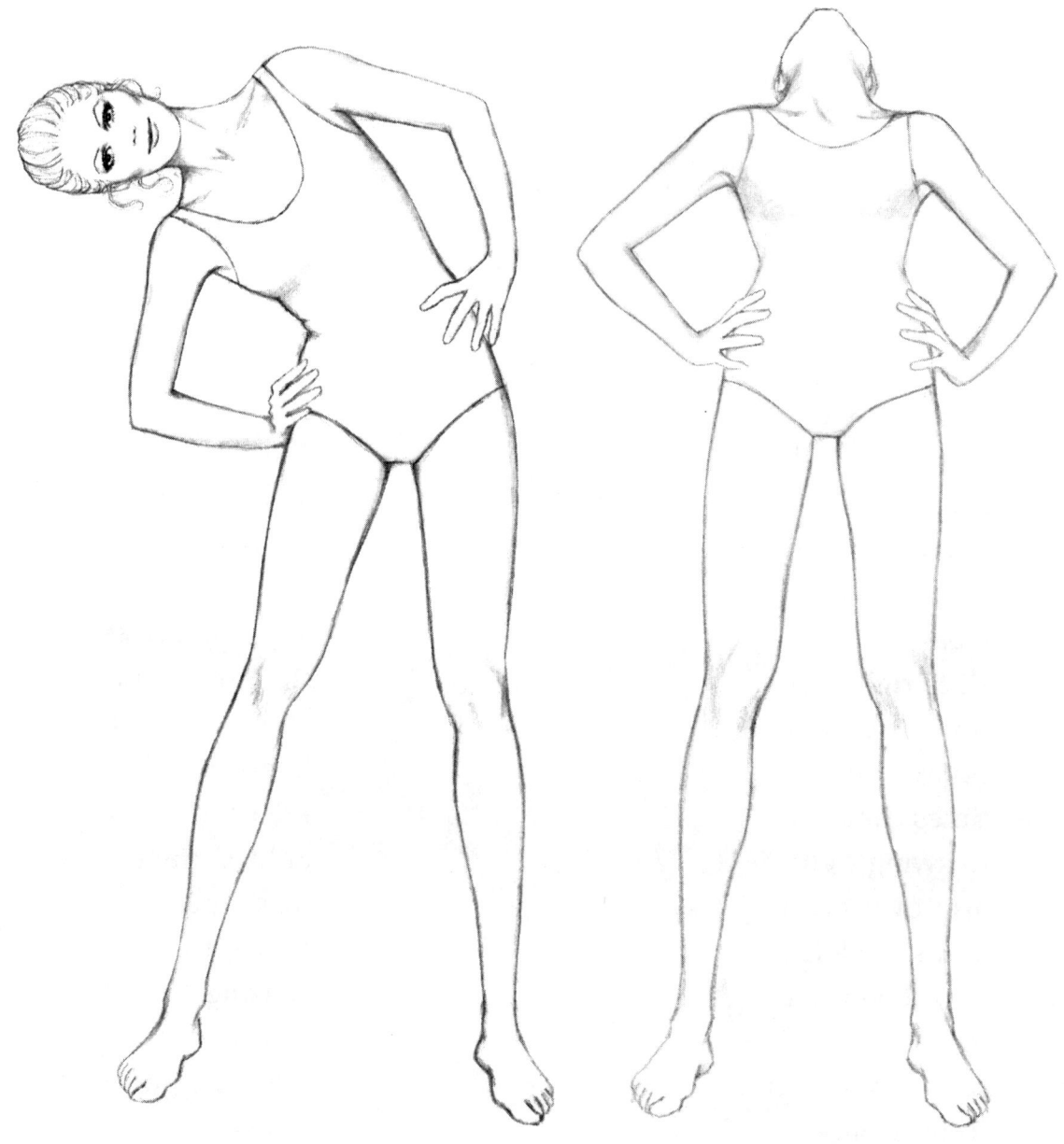

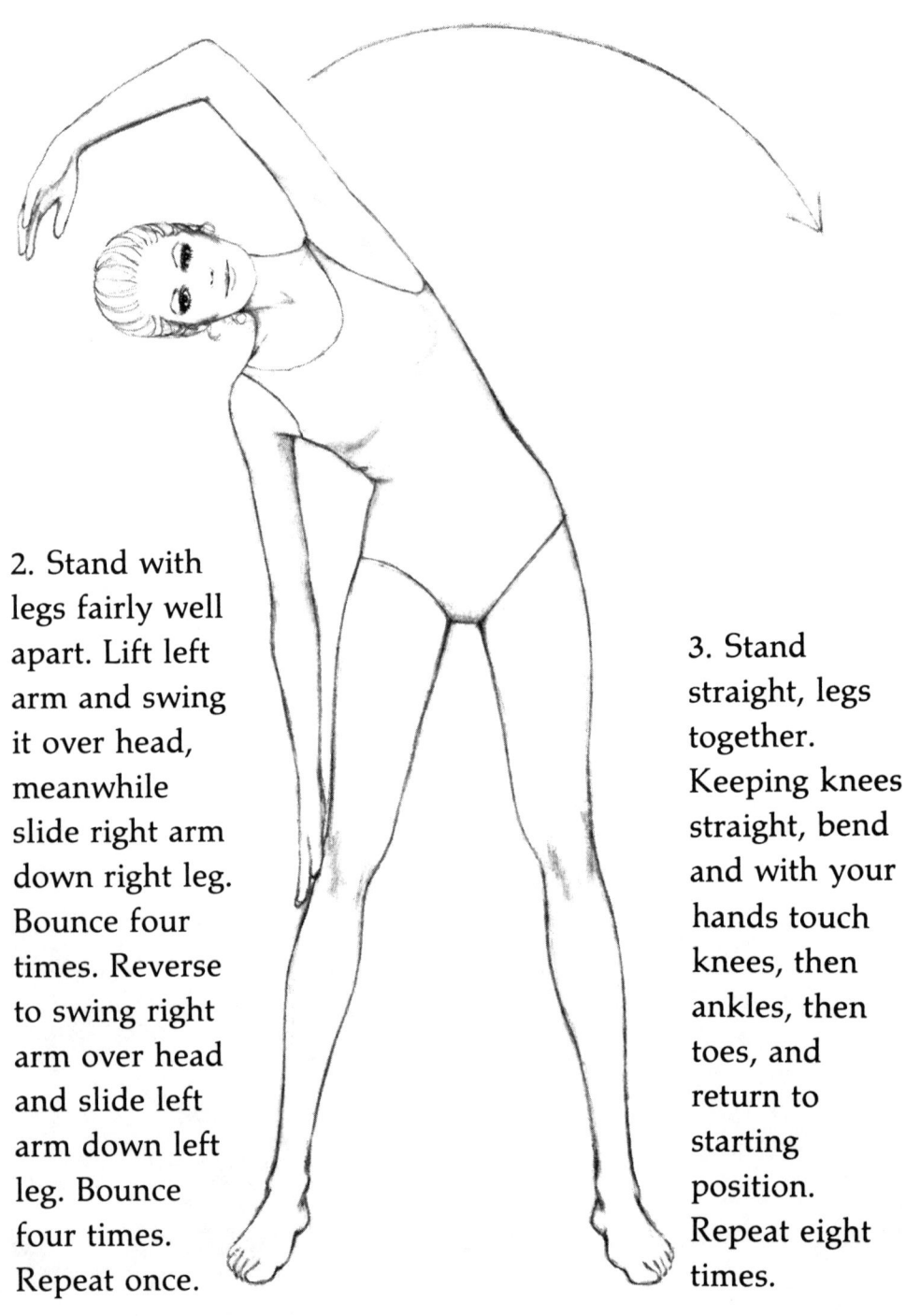

2. Stand with legs fairly well apart. Lift left arm and swing it over head, meanwhile slide right arm down right leg. Bounce four times. Reverse to swing right arm over head and slide left arm down left leg. Bounce four times. Repeat once.

3. Stand straight, legs together. Keeping knees straight, bend and with your hands touch knees, then ankles, then toes, and return to starting position. Repeat eight times.

ABDOMEN

1. Lie on back on floor, head resting on hands, knees flexed with feet close to buttocks. Press small of back flat onto floor, and suck in abdomen. Hold for 20 seconds, breathing normally throughout exercise.
2. Work your way up to 20 sit-ups.
3. Lie on back with palms on floor beside buttocks. Slowly lift legs together to an upright position, perpendicular to floor. Slowly lower to three inches above floor, hold for count of six, and return. Repeat twice, and work up to six in succession.
4. Lie on back, knees flexed, and clasp head. Sit up slowly, and touch right elbow to left knee. Return to lying position. Reverse, with left elbow touching right knee. Repeat four times.

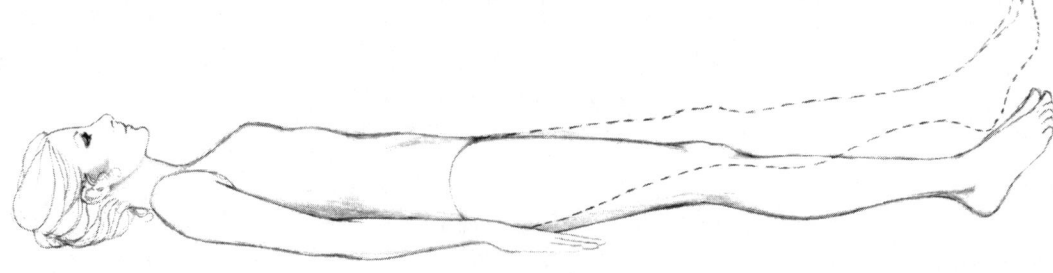

BUTTOCKS

1. Sitting up, legs extended straight out in front, bounce on alternating buttocks to count of 10.
2. Sitting up, legs extended straight out in front, "walk" forward by wiggling on buttocks from side to side for a count of 20. Walk backward for a count of 20.
3. Stand and alternately squeeze and relax buttocks for 20 counts.

THIGHS, LEGS, AND ANKLES

1. Stand straight; hold on to steady chair with left hand. Hug right knee to chest (or as close as possible to chest), and rotate right foot in a complete circle four times. Reverse to other knee rotating left foot.
2. Walk on tiptoes.
3. Lie on stomach, forehead resting on hands. Keep legs straight. Slowly raise right leg, toes pointed, about a foot off floor. Hold for three seconds. Slowly lower. Repeat for left leg. Repeat three times working up to six times.

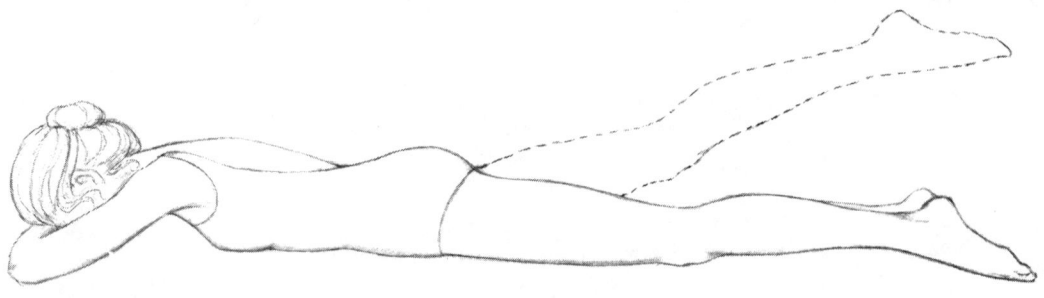

Sport Exercise

To receive maximum benefits from exercise you must work out. Make your heart beat faster, lungs pump harder, and get your blood circulation going from head to toe. This can only be accomplished with vigorous exercise. Do your spot exercises three times weekly; then twice a week take part in one of the following activities; all are great overall toners. Start off slowly and work up to a fast, long pace.

JOGGING	VOLLEYBALL	SKATING
●	●	●
TENNIS	SOCCER	GOLF
●	●	●
JUMPING ROPE	CYCLING	HIKING
●	●	●
RACQUETBALL	SWIMMING	HORSEBACK RIDING
●	●	●
BASKETBALL	SKIING	DISCO DANCING
●		
SQUASH		

Keep challenging your body and stretch yourself. For example, hike uphill, cycle for long distances, swim an extra lap.

Dance is not really a sport, but is just as strenuous and builds and tones the body.

If you have any doubts about your physical condition, consult a doctor before participating in these activities.

Tips
- Warm up with the "Hymn to the Sun" exercise, stretching, and jumping jacks.
- Cool down with legs propped up and a large glass of water, a tepid shower, or a cool bath.
- Join a gym or health club for encouragement.
- Wear athletic shoes for jogging and other sports.
- Wear a bra if breasts are medium to large size.

WHEN TO SEE A DOCTOR

When you have doubts about your physical condition or not, practice preventive medicine. See doctors for checkups on a regular basis and you'll decrease the need of having to see them on an emergency basis. The point of going for checkups is to permit the trained professional to notice the beginning of a problem before it becomes an obvious problem to you. Every half year, consult a dentist and a gynecologist; every two years see an opthamologist and a good general practitioner or internist for a complete physical. And, of course, if you suspect any problems, see a doctor.

THE RELAXATION EXERCISE

Tension usually distorts the features with tight lips, furrowed brows, and nervous twitches. Learning to relax is good for your appearance as well as your emotional state. Enjoy this exercise, and remember that when you are relaxing, time is not being wasted. You are revitalizing and refreshing yourself.

1. Sit down comfortably. Better yet, lie down with legs slightly elevated.
2. Breathe deeply
3. Clear your mind of thoughts.
4. Concentrate on relaxing words: calm, tranquil, serene, peaceful.
5. Envision yourself as a calm, tranquil, serene person.
6. Remain in position for five to 10 minutes. Repeat as often as desired.

SLEEP

Sleep is essential for beauty. All the concealer in the world won't hide the dark shadows, bad complexion, and general lack of vitality that a steady routine of insufficient sleep brings on. The amount of nightly sleep each individual requires may vary anywhere from five to nine hours. Learn how many hours you need to function best, and learn to say no to making commitments that will interfere with your getting that amount.

If you have occasional bouts of insomnia, the old-fashioned remedies of taking a warm bath and drinking warm milk work, as heat and calcium are both muscle relaxants. At least an hour before you retire, create a peaceful environment and get ready for bed. Half an hour before bedtime, practice the relaxation exercise to eliminate accumulated tension. Once in bed, lie on the side of the body you don't normally lie on to sleep. Do not roll over when the urge to do so first hits. Force yourself to remain in this position for as long as you can. Eventually you'll just have to roll over to your normal sleep position and should drift off to sleep right away.

A WORD ON COSMETIC SURGERY

If you read this book thoroughly, and put into practice the techniques and tips for good health care and cosmetic applications, you could end up looking and feeling so good that the idea of surgery for you would be superfluous. Some beauty problems are so severe or so disturbing to the person who has them, however, that no amount of exercise, beauty management or makeup will diminish or correct the flaw. Surgery can be considered as an alternative to futile efforts at camouflaging the problem, but do keep in mind the seriousness of this particular process in a beauty makeover.

First, it is surgery, with all the risks that are a part of any major surgery. Second, it is often a painful and not easily altered change. Third, it is quite expensive. If you do desire cosmetic surgery, here is a brief explanation of the most common types:

- Nose (rhinoplasty): Noses can be shortened or straightened, bumps removed, nostrils reshaped, bridges rebuilt.
- Eyes (blepharoplasty): Bags and drooping lids can be corrected.
- Face lift (rhytidectomy): Wrinkles, folds, and lines are corrected. Lasts from five to 10 years.
- Ears (otoplasty): Large ears are made smaller; protruding ears are corrected.
- Chin (mentoplasty): Receding chins are built up; protruding jaws are decreased.
- Breasts (mammoplasty): Breasts are enlarged or decreased.
- Thigh and buttocks lift: Excess fat can be removed.

Cosmetic surgery can also rectify a variety of skin problems, including the removal of birthmarks or a deeply scarred surface on the skin.

Make sure you select a reliable physician. Check with your family doctor or the best hospital around for a recommended surgeon. As with all serious medical considerations, get two opinions.

THE RIGHT TIMES

Now that you have taken stock of your hair, skin, figure, and features and determined what techniques and regimens you need, it's time to get organized. Two key elements in any beauty makeover are organization and routine. By organizing your tools and equipment, you can free time normally spent in search of these things for other activities. Set up a routine that includes all the procedures you need to follow by consulting our lists below and making your own personalized plan, one that you can refer to again and again until it becomes a habit.

DAILY

Choose foods from the
Basic Four.

●

Bathe or shower (don't
forget lotions).

●

Wash face (two or three times daily).

●

Use toner, moisturizer (two or three times daily).

●

Make up.

●

Check eyebrows; tweeze if necessary.

●

Brush teeth (two times daily).

●

Floss.

●

Shampoo if necessary.

●

Condition hair if necessary.

●

Check posture.

•

Use deodorant.

•

Use fragrance.

WEEKLY

Clean face with scrubbing agent (once or twice weekly).

•

Apply facial mask.

•

Give yourself a manicure.

•

Spot exercise (three times weekly).

•

Sport exercise (twice weekly).

•

Launder and dry-clean clothes.

●

Check clothes for repairs.

SEMIMONTHLY

Facial steam.

●

Pedicure.

MONTHLY

Put deep, penetrating conditioner on hair.

●

Visit hairdresser (every four to six weeks).

EVERY SIX MONTHS

See dentist.

●

See gynecologist.

●

EVERY TWO YEARS

See opthalmologist.

●

Go for routine physical.

●

Make lists of your own personal priorities under these same categories.

Daily	Weekly	
Morning	Monday	Saturday
●	●	●
Midday	Tuesday	Sunday
●	●	●
Evening	Wednesday	*Semimonthly and monthly*
●	●	*Every Six Months*
	Thursday	*Every Two Years*
	●	
	Friday	
	●	

PERFECTING NEW TECHNIQUES

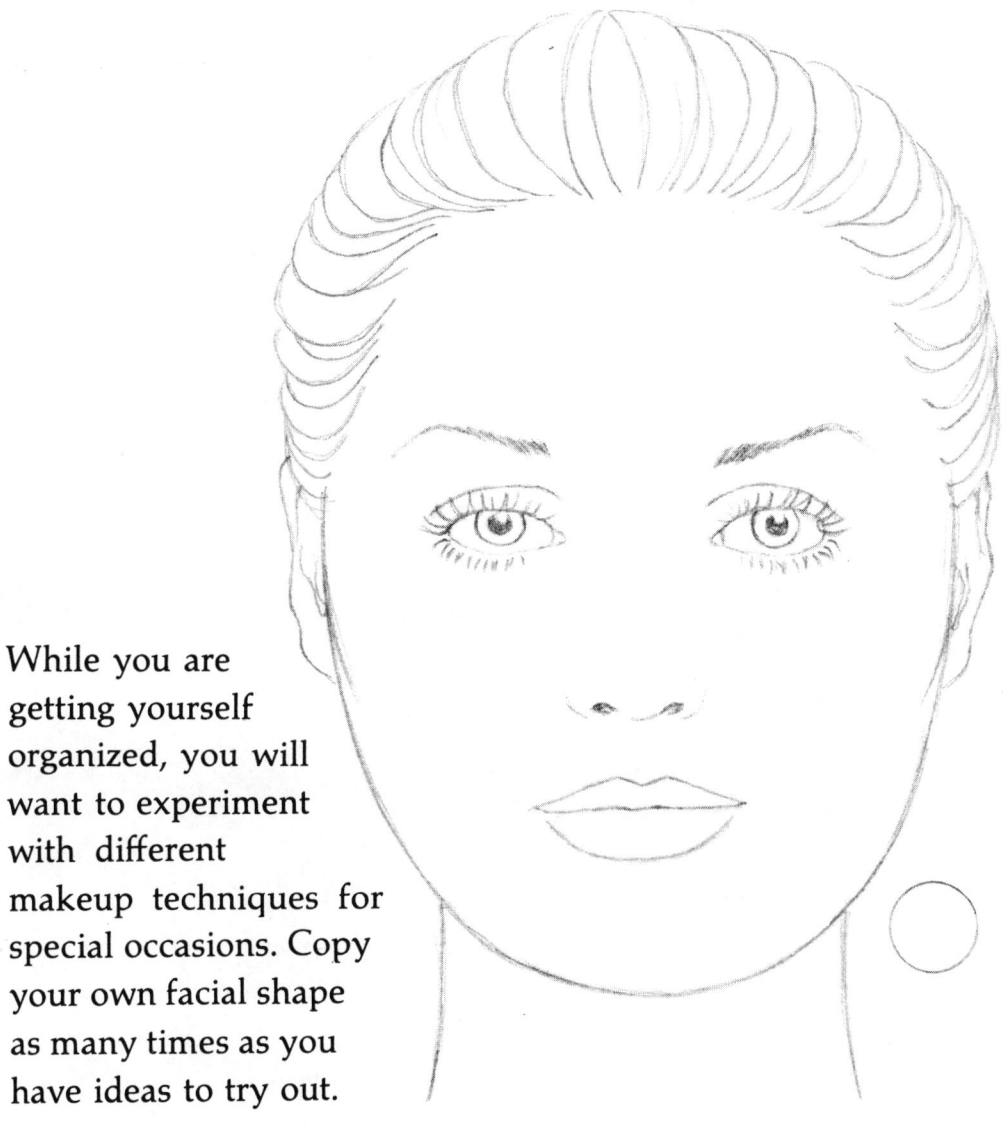

While you are getting yourself organized, you will want to experiment with different makeup techniques for special occasions. Copy your own facial shape as many times as you have ideas to try out.

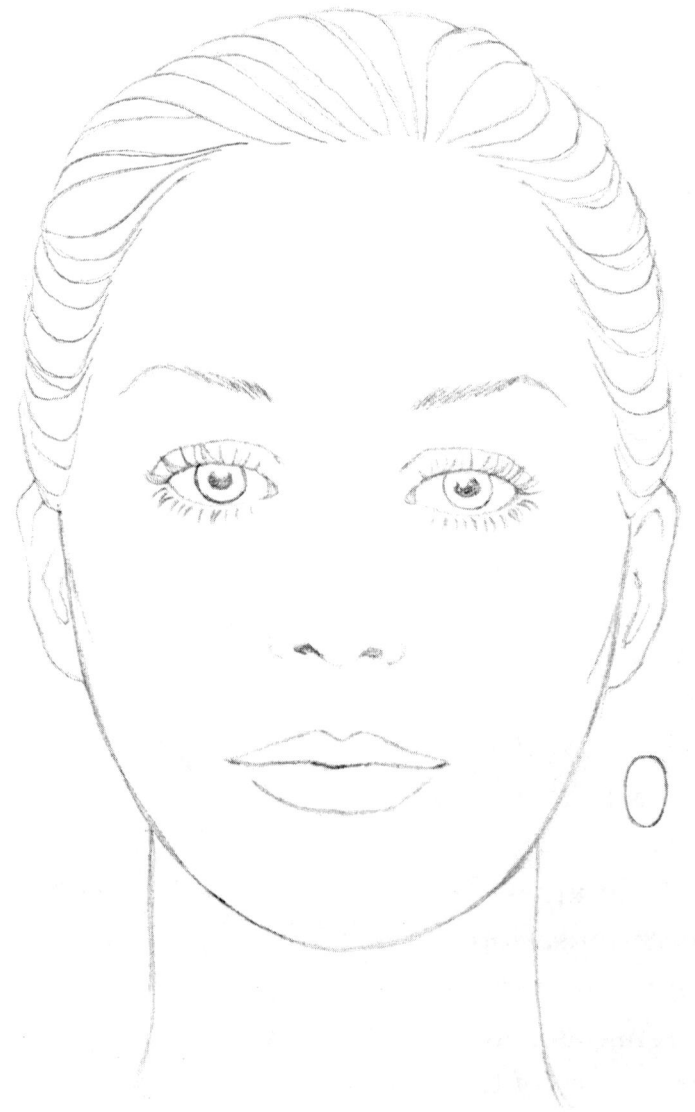

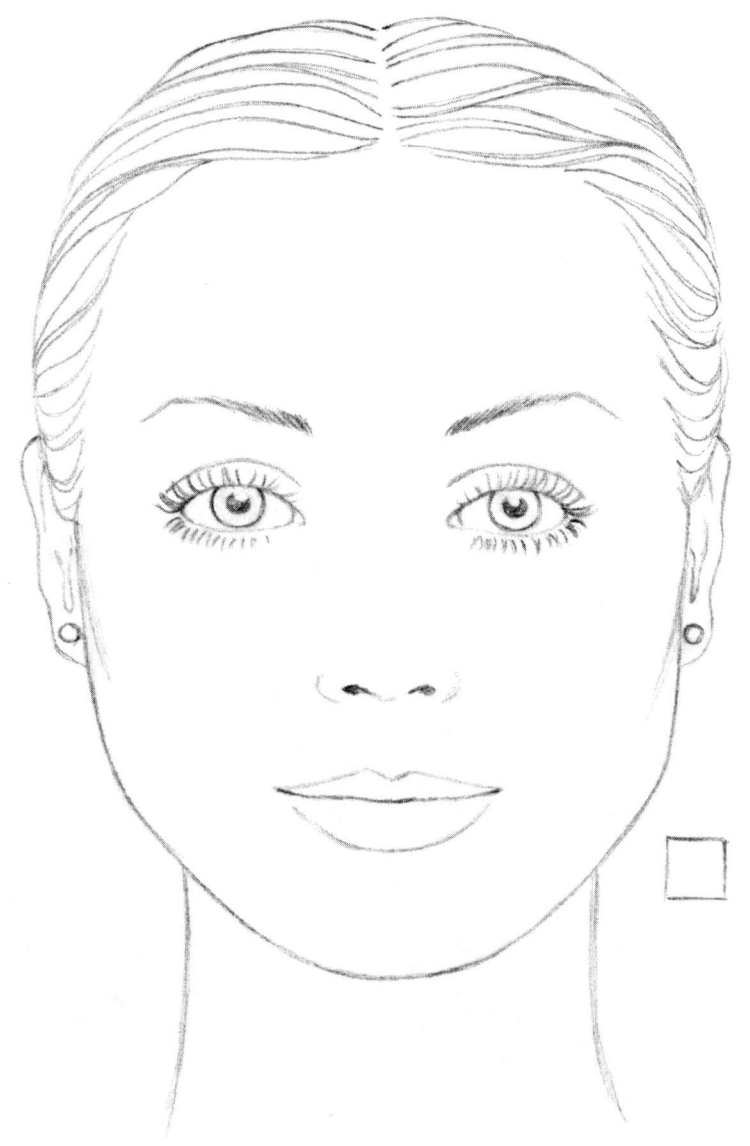

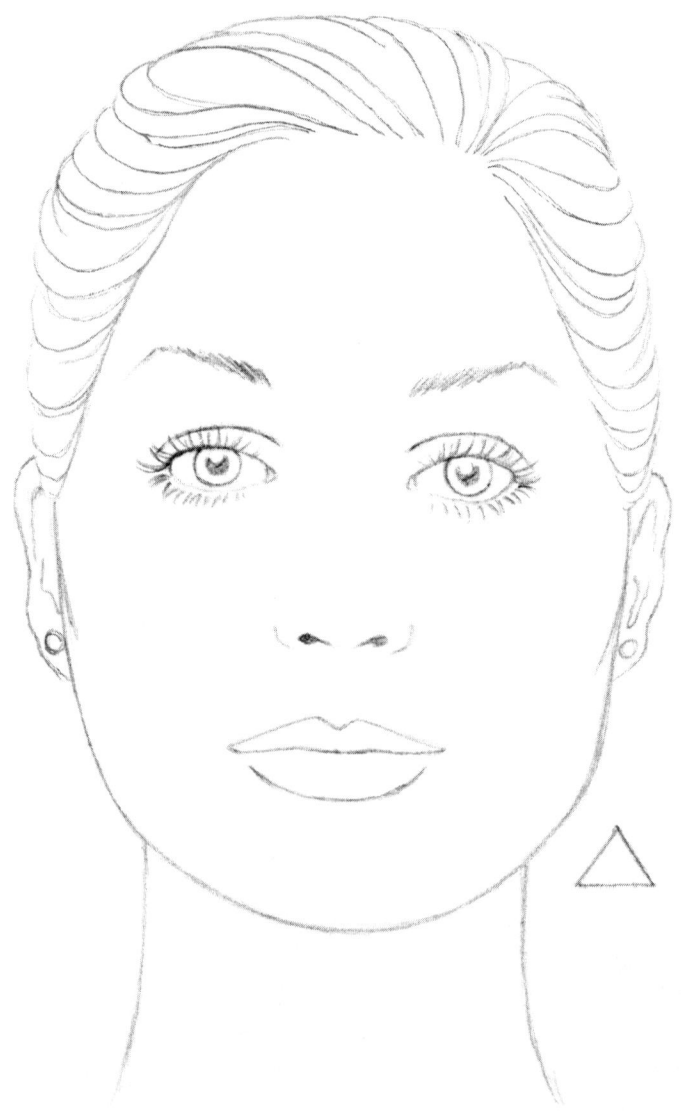

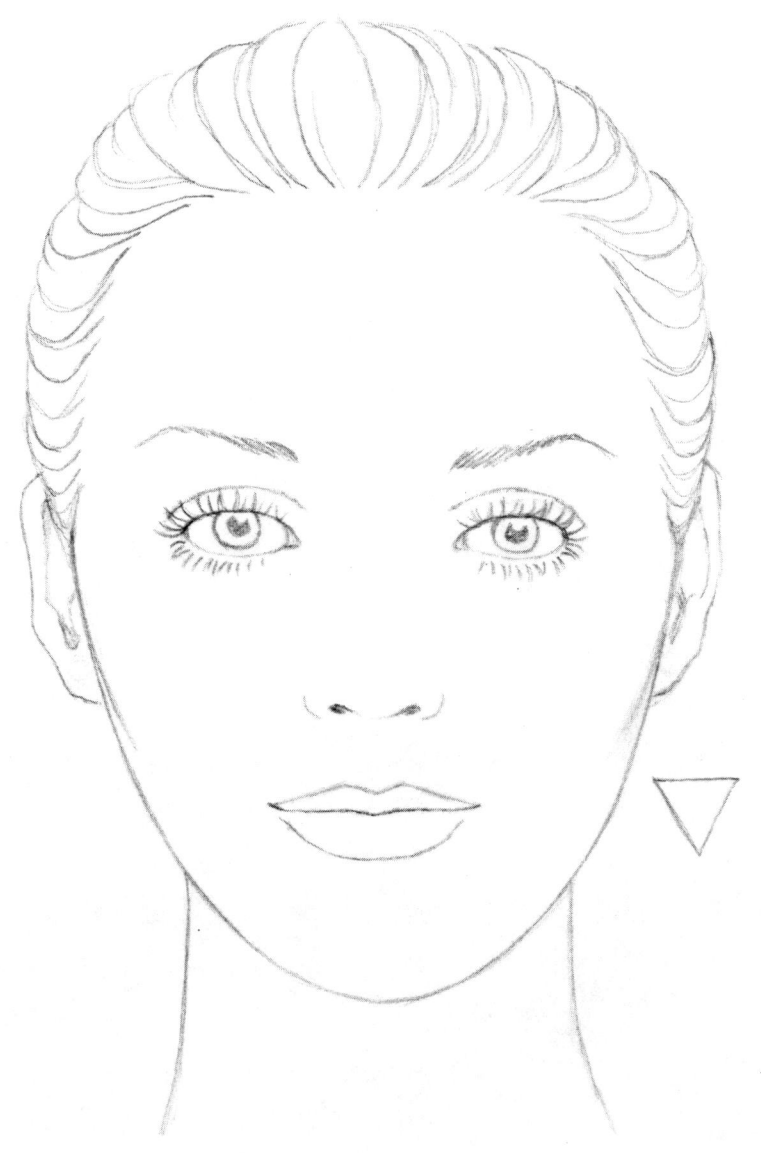

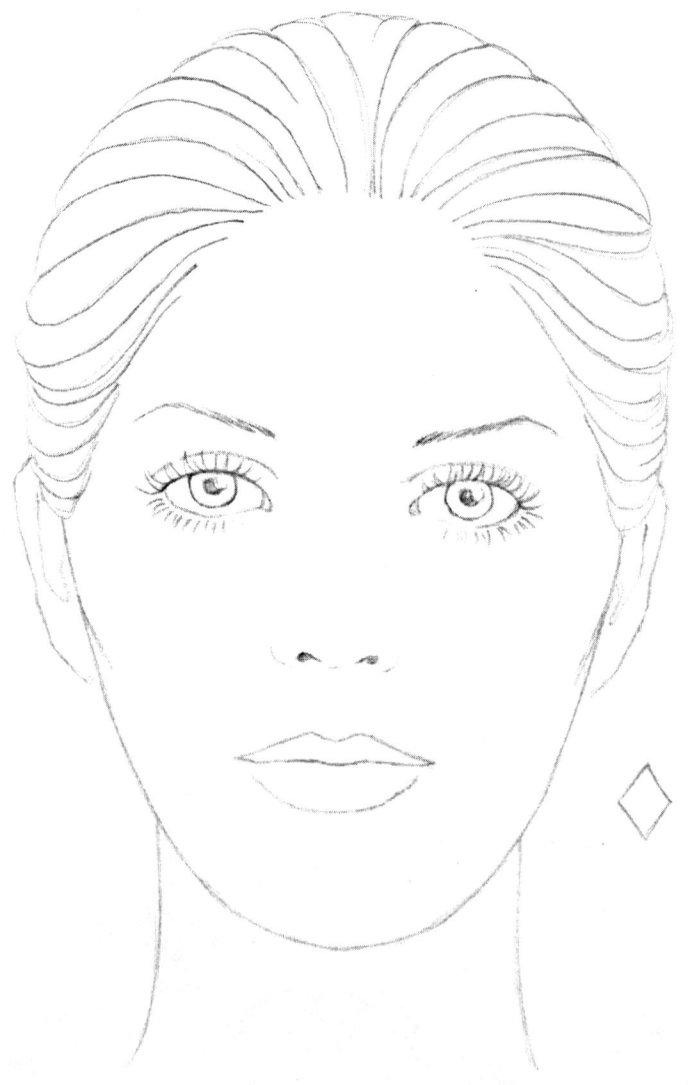

CONCLUSION

Scheduling a routine for yourself may be the end of our book, but it is a new beginning for you.

By completing this book, you have taken the first step toward making yourself over. You've learned which methods and materials are necessary to maximize your beauty assets and minimize your less attractive liabilities. Now you know the techniques involved and you know that becoming a more beautiful, healthier woman is not a complicated process. Review the information, experiment, devise a program, and stay with it.

You will fulfill your beauty potential.

Terms to Remember

ALLERGY TEST. Test for skin sensitivity. Rub substance in question on inner arm, cover with bandage and wait 24 hours. If no reaction, product is safe for your use.

ANTIPERSPIRANT. A product used to decrease wetness as well as to stop odor.

ASTRINGENT. Strongest form of toner, used to close pores, remove dead cells, restore proper pH to skin.

BASIC FOUR. Four groups of food from which you must eat daily to obtain all necessary nutrients. See section on Body Tonics.

CHEEK BRUSH. A brush specifically designed for use with a powder form of cheek color.

COLOGNE. A mild form of fragrance, without the staying power of perfume.

CONDITIONER. A product applied to the hair to improve or stabilize its condition; may be rinsed out or left on.

CONTOURER. The use of a dark foundation or product specially formulated to decrease the intensity of a specific facial area.

CREAM RINSE. A product applied to hair after shampooing and then rinsed out which leaves a light film to make hair shiny, more manageable, and easier to comb.

CURLING IRON. An electrically heated rod or wand used to do spot curls or entire head of curls.

DEODORANT. A product used to minimize offensive odor.

DEPILATORY. Solution with strong chemical to remove unwanted hair.

DEPILATRON. Method of removing unwanted hair by sending an electrical current into the hair root by tweezers.

EAU DE PARFUM. Least concentrated form of fragrance, sometimes called "eau fraiche" or "splash."

ELECTRIC ROLLERS. A set of rollers heated electrically to produce curls in five minutes.

ELECTROLYSIS. Method of removing unwanted hair by sending a tiny electrical current into hair root via insertion of a very fine needle.

FACIAL DIRECTIONALS. Proper direction of movement when applying substances to face in order to avoid wrinkling, etc.

FACIAL MASK. A method of refreshing and tightening facial skin by permitting various substances to dry on face and be removed with water or by peeling off.

FACIAL STEAM. A method of steaming open pores to achieve a deep cleansing effect.

FOUNDATION. A cream or liquid used as a base for makeup.

FRESHENER. The mildest form of toner, a specially formulated lotion used to close pores, remove dead cells, restore proper pH to skin.

HENNA. A temporary dye applied to the hair which fades with washing; available in natural, red, brown, or black.

HIGHLIGHTER. The use of a white or light-colored foundation to increase the intensity of a specific facial area.

"HYMN TO THE SUN". Yoga movements used to warm up before or cool down after exercising. See section on exercise.

LIP BRUSH. A brush made from natural or man-made fibers used to outline the shape of the lips.

LIP GLOSS. A clear, shiny base for the lips; may be worn alone or over a lipstick.

LOOFAH. Dried shell of plants; resembles a sponge; used as a skin scrubber.

MANICURE. Procedure of hand care concentrating on fingernails, their upkeep and polish.

MOISTURIZER. Cream or lotion solution specially formulated to maintain moisture on surface of skin. Usually used for face and neck area only.

NUTRIENTS. Basic food substances that provide essential nourishment; most necessary are proteins, carbohydrates, fats, vitamins, minerals, water.

PEDICURE. Procedure of foot care concentrating on toenails, their polish and upkeep.

PERFUME. The strongest form of fragrance.

pH (potential of hydrogen). The degree of acidity or alkalinity in a substance, assigned with a number from zero to 14.

PUMICE STONE. Rough, grainy stone used to slough dead skin, calluses, corns.

QUALITY OF HAIR. Refers to the diameter of the hair shaft: fine, medium, coarse.

QUANTITY OF HAIR. Refers to the amount of hair on the scalp; thin, normal, thick.

RELAXATION EXERCISE. Procedure of relaxation effective any time.

SACHET. A fragrance usually sold as a powder to scent clothes; available in cream for use on the body.

SPORT EXERCISE. Activities other than calisthenics (spot exercises); they generally speed up body processes, are good overall body toners.

SPOT EXERCISES. Calisthenics; organized movements to tone specific muscles.

SUNSCREEN. Preparation for use on the skin that screens out some tanning rays.

TONER. General term for a specially formulated lotion used to close pores, remove dead cells, and restore proper pH to skin; also specific term for the form of this lotion of medium strength, when the strongest form is called an astringent and the weakest a freshener.

UNDERTONER. Lotion used underneath foundation to neutralize or offset skin's uneven tones and complement the surface skin color.

Readings for Health

The Complete Book of Running, by James F. Fixx. New York: Random House, 1977.

Nicole Ronsard's No-Excuse Exercise Guide, by Nicole Ronsard. New York: William Morrow & Co., 1976.

Our Bodies, Our Selves, by Boston Women's Health Book Collective. New York: Simon and Schuster, Inc., 1976.

Nutrition Almanac, by John D. Kirschmann. New York: McGraw-Hill, Inc., 1975.

Let's Eat Right to Keep Fit, by Adelle Davis. New York: Harcourt, Brace & World, 1954.

Richard Hittleman's Introduction to Yoga, by Richard Hittleman. New York: Bantam Books, 1969.